Key Concepts in
Healthcare
Education

The SAGE Key Concepts series provides students with accessible and authoritative knowledge of the essential topics in a variety of disciplines. Cross-referenced throughout, the format encourages critical evaluation through understanding. Written by experienced and respected academics, the books are indispensable study aids and guides to comprehension.

ANNETTE MCINTOSH, JANICE GIDMAN AND ELIZABETH MASON-WHITEHEAD

Key Concepts in
Healthcare
Education

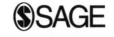

Los Angeles | London | New Delhi
Singapore | Washington DC

SAGE Publications Ltd
1 Oliver's Yard
55 City Road
London EC1Y 1SP

SAGE Publications Inc.
2455 Teller Road
Thousand Oaks, California 91320

SAGE Publications India Pvt Ltd
B 1/I 1 Mohan Cooperative Industrial Area
Mathura Road
New Delhi 110 044

SAGE Publications Asia-Pacific Pte Ltd
33 Pekin Street #02-01
Far East Square
Singapore 048763

Library of Congress Control Number: 2009943438

British Library Cataloguing in Publication data

A catalogue record for this book is available from the British Library

ISBN 978-1-84920-009-7
ISBN 978-1-84920-010-3 (pbk)

Typeset by C&M Digitals (P) Ltd, Chennai, India
Printed in India at Replika Press Pvt Ltd
Printed on paper from sustainable resources

To Nina Sinclair

contents

contents

key concepts in
healthcare education

contents

list of tables

key concepts in
healthcare education

x

list of figures

list of contributors

EDITORS

Annette McIntosh, PhD, BSc, Cert Ed, Dip CNE, FHEA, RGN, SCM, RNT, RCNT is the Associate Dean, Learning and Teaching, in the Faculty of Health and Social Care at the University of Chester, UK

Janice Gidman, PhD, MEd, BSc (Hons), PGCE, FHEA, ONC, RN is a Senior Teaching Fellow in the Faculty of Health and Social Care at the University of Chester, UK

Elizabeth, Mason-Whitehead PhD, BA (Hons), HV, PGDE, ONC, SRN, SCM is Professor of Social and Health Care in the Faculty of Health and Social Care at the University of Chester, UK

CONTRIBUTORS

Nicola Andrew, Prof D, MN, PGCE, FHEA, RN is a Senior Lecturer in the School of Health at Glasgow Caledonian University, UK

Margaret Andrews, MSc, BSc, FHEA, RN, RCNT, RNT is Pro-Vice Chancellor (Students) and Professor at Canterbury Christ Church University, UK

Julie Bailey-McHale, MSc, PG Dip Ed, BSc (Hons), RMN is a Senior Lecturer and Programme Leader in Mental Health in the Education and Training Centre, Isle of Man

Peter Bradshaw, MA, BNurs., RN, RMN, RHV, RNT is Professor of Health Care Policy at the University of Huddersfield, UK

Ann Bryan, MSc, Cert Ed, FHEA, ADM, RGN, RM, HV, RMT is Head of Community and Child Health in the Faculty of Health and Social Care at the University of Chester, UK

Elisabeth Clark, PhD, BA (Hons) is the Deputy Director of the Open University – Royal College of Nursing Strategic Alliance, in the Faculty of Health and Social Care, The Open University, UK

Helen Cooper, PhD, BNurs., PGCHE, FHEA, RGN, RHV, DN Cert. is Professor of Community and Child Health in the Faculty of Health and Social Care at the University of Chester, UK

key concepts in healthcare education

Chris Cox is Director of Legal Services, Royal College of Nursing

Kay Currie, PhD, PGCert., MN, BSc (Nursing), RN, RNT is Reader in Nursing in the School of Health at Glasgow Caledonian University, UK

Wendy Fiander, MA Information Studies, BSc (Hons), Member of the Chartered Institute of Information Professionals (MCLIP), FHEA is the Deputy Director of Learning and Information Services at the University of Chester, UK

Sandra Flynn, MSc, BA (Hons), RGN, ONC, DPSN is Nurse Consultant in Orthopaedics in the Countess of Chester Hospital, Chester, UK

Jane Fox, PhD, MPhil, MSc, BA, Cert Ed/RNT, DN, ONC, SRN is Development Manager, Skills for Health, UK

Bernadette Gartside, MA (supporting Dyslexic Learners), PG Dip (Dyslexia and Literacy), Cert Ed, associate Member of the British Dyslexia Association (AMBDA) is an Academic Skills Tutor (Dyslexia Specialist) at the University of Chester, UK

Morag Gray, PhD, MN, Dip CNE, Cert. Ed, FHEA, RGN, RCNT, RNT is Professor, Associate Dean (Academic Development) and Senior Teaching Fellow in the Faculty of Health, Life and Social Sciences at Edinburgh Napier University, UK

Karen Holland, MSc, BSc (Hons), Cert Ed, RGN, RNT is Research Fellow (Evidence Based Nurse Education Innovation) in the School of Nursing & Midwifery at the University of Salford, UK

Moira Hulme, PhD, MEd, MA, MA, BSc (Hons), PGCE is a Lecturer in Educational Research in the Faculty of Education at the University of Glasgow, UK

Rob Hulme, MA, BA (Hons), Cert Ed is Professor of Education and Director of the Research Unit for Trans-professionalism in the Public Services, Faculty of Education and Children's Services at the University of Chester, UK

Annette Jinks, PhD, MA, BA, RN, NDN is Professor of Nursing in the Faculty of Health at Edge Hill University, UK

Sue Lillyman, MA (Ed), BSc (Nursing) RN, RM, DPSN, PGCE, RNT is a Senior Lecturer in Allied Health Sciences in the Institute of Health and Society at the University of Worcester, UK

Andrew Lovell, PhD, BA (Hons), Cert Ed, RNLD is a Reader in Learning Disabilities in the Faculty of Health and Social Care at the University of Chester, UK

Jean Mannix, MEd, BA (Hons) SCPHN, RN, HV is Deputy Head of Community and Child Health in the Faculty of Health and Social Care at the University of Chester, UK

Dorothy Marriss, PhD, MA, BEd (Hons), Cert Ed, Dip Nurs, FHEA, ONC, SRN, RNT, RCNT is Deputy Vice-Chancellor (Academic) at the University of Chester, UK

Tom Mason, PhD, BSc(Hons), FHEA, RMN, RNMH, RGN is Professor and Head of Mental Health and Learning Disabilities in the Faculty of Health and Social Care at the University of Chester, UK

Jill McCarthy, PhD, MSc, MA, BEd (Hons), Cert Ed, FHEA, RGN, DN Cert, RNT is a Senior Lecturer and e-learning co-ordinator in the Faculty of Health and Social Care at the University of Chester, UK

Andrea McLaughlin, MEd, Cert Ed., FHEA, RGN, RM, ADM is Head of Midwifery and Reproductive Health in the Faculty of Health and Social Care at the University of Chester, UK

Lyz Moore, BSc(Hons), PGCert HE, RN is a Lecturer in the Education and Training Centre, Isle of Man

Dianne Phipps, MA, PGCE, RNMH is Deputy Head of Mental Health and Learning Disabilities in the Faculty of Health and Social Care at the University of Chester, UK

Tracey Proctor-Childs, MA (Education), BSc (Hons) Nursing, Dip Nurs, RN, RM is Deputy Head (Learning and Teaching) of the School of Nursing and Midwifery at the University of Plymouth, UK

Linda Proudfoot, MPhil, BA (Nursing Studies), RN, DN is a Practice Educator /Lecturer in the School of Health at Glasgow Caledonian University, UK

Mike Thomas, PhD, MA, BNurs., CertEd., FHEA, RMN, RNT is Professor of Mental Health and Executive Dean of the Faculty of Health and Social Care at the University of Chester, UK

Maureen Wilkins, MEd, RGN, RCNT, RNT is Head of Professional Development and Allied Health Care in the Faculty of Health and Social Care at the University of Chester, UK

Julie Williams, MSc, DipHE, DPSN, MHS (cert), PGCE, RGN, RNT is Head of Pre-registration Nursing in the Faculty of Health and Social Care at the University of Chester, UK

Terry Williams, MBA, Certificate in Social Work, Certificate in Social Work Management is the Co-ordinator and Development Worker in the Forum for Carers and Users of Services (FOCUS) in Cheshire and Merseyside, UK

Jan Woodhouse, MEd, PGDE, BN (Hons), Dip N, RGN, OND, FETC is a Senior Lecturer in the Faculty of Health and Social Care at the University of Chester, UK

Aidan Worsley, MPhil, MA Social Work (inc CQSW), BSc (Hons), Practice Teaching Award, FHEA is Professor and Head of Social Work at the University of Central Lancashire, UK

CASE STUDY CONTRIBUTORS

Mark Hellaby, BSc(Hons), RODP, RN is an MEd student and Clinical Skills/ Simulation Facilitator at Warrington and Halton Hospitals NHS Foundation Trust, Cheshire, UK

Janine Upton, MSc, PGDE, RGN, ONC is a Senior Lecturer, Pre-registration Nursing, in the Faculty of Health and Social Care at the University of Chester, UK

acknowledgements

There are many people the editors wish to acknowledge in the development and production of this book.

Our thanks and gratitude go to:

- the lecturing staff of the Faculty of Health and Social Care, University of Chester, for their help in identifying the key concepts for educators in healthcare;
- the staff at Sage Publications who supported the premise of this book and offered invaluable guidance throughout the process, from conception to publication, particularly Zoe Elliot-Fawcett, Emma Paterson Alison Poyner and Katie Forsythe;
- the authors, for their expert contributions;
- our partners, Peter, Steve and Tom, for their forbearance and support in this endeavour.

key concepts in
healthcare education

editors' preface

This book presents 40 concepts for educators in healthcare, providing a comprehensive overview of the key theories, literature, drivers and practical considerations involved in educating in the healthcare professions in the 21st century.

There are many involved in healthcare who have a responsibility for education as part of their role. While this can include promoting health through educating service users, carers and the general public, this text is primarily concerned with those educating students of healthcare at all levels, from pre-qualifying programmes through to doctoral levels of study.

The current context of healthcare education requires that all individuals involved in the endeavour have a thorough grounding in a broad range of operational and theoretical concepts, alongside the skills to teach, support and inspire students in both educational and practice settings. To be effective in the art of educating requires an understanding of the contextual factors and drivers at three levels: macro, meso and micro.

The macro level incorporates aspects such as political and economic drivers in healthcare and in education. These currently include a quality assurance approach to educating in healthcare which is based on targets and standards. This has led to corresponding changes in the aims of professional education programmes which have become increasingly competence-based. It is evident that there are potential tensions between outcome-driven curricula, which have to conform to rigid professional standards, and the need for professionals to respond effectively to the constantly changing environments of healthcare. Contemporary government and professional policies also promote integrated services, interagency working and increased public involvement in all aspects of healthcare services. This requires healthcare programmes to incorporate interprofessional learning opportunities and to include service users in programme planning, recruitment, delivery and evaluation. External agencies also influence culture by exercising indirect control over institutions, with increasing levels of accountability required for teaching and research. Best practice is identified and sustained through quality assurance and enhancement. The challenges, opportunities and issues for staff development are mainly a response to these initiatives, with healthcare educators required to keep up to date with current policies and teaching methods and accept responsibility for change. The meso context in healthcare education concerns the institutional or organisational level. The extensive literature related to healthcare education highlights potential tensions between the need for practitioners to be fit for practice at the point of qualification, maintaining the interests of public safety, whilst adopting the ethos of higher education to empower students throughout their studies. Similar challenges exist with qualified professionals, required to engage in lifelong learning and studying as part-time students while holding down demanding jobs. Indeed, many full-time educators in higher education find themselves in this position, with the expectation that all lecturers will have doctoral level qualifications and be research active, alongside maintaining clinical and professional credibility.

There are many aspects involved in the context of the micro level of health-care education, that is, all things concerned with the development, planning and management of educational provision for students. Professional education programmes in healthcare adopt humanistic, student-centred approaches and incorporate both academic and practice-based learning and assessment. Recent professional and quality assurance requirements have strengthened the emphasis on practice-based learning and assessment within many pro-grammes. However, tensions can be identified in relation to several compet-ing agendas, for example, professional competence and student empowerment, professional roles and interprofessional learning and the relationships between service users and professionals.

Clearly then, educating in healthcare requires consideration of a myriad of concepts, some theoretical and some operational, that interlink and weave together to form a theoretical network to support educators. This book sets out to bring these together for readers and is relevant to anyone with a teach-ing responsibility in healthcare. For those starting out in education, be it as lecturers within an Higher Education Institution, educators or mentors in practice or, indeed, pre-qualifying students addressing the teaching elements inherent in the role of healthcare professionals, these key concepts provide a sound base from which to develop the knowledge and skills to become an effective and competent educator in healthcare. For those more experienced in the education for, and of, health care professions, including managers, this book offers support for the essential pursuit of ongoing personal and profes-sional development.

Each entry is written by an author with expertise in the field, drawing together the salient points for the reader, underpinned by research and litera-ture and a practical application of the concept. The text is arranged alpha-betically for easy referencing and each chapter provides a comprehensive, yet succinct, account of a key concept and features:

- a definition.
- list of key points.
- discussion of the main elements of the concept.
- a case study to illustrate the application and usefulness of the theory to real world situations of educational practice.
- a conclusion.
- cross-references to other concepts, to facilitate linkages to be made.
- some suggestions for further reading.

This book, therefore, provides an overview of all the key concepts required in being an effective educator in healthcare in any context. Ensuring a sound educational experience for students is a significant responsibility and educators are required to have and develop the knowledge, skills and expertise to facilitate learning, often in the dual learning environments of academic and practice settings and in the broad context in which healthcare education takes place.

Annette McIntosh, Janice Gidman and Elizabeth Mason-Whitehead
Chester, UK
October 2009

1 academic staff development

Dorothy Marriss

DEFINITION

Staff development is a sufficiently complex concept to defy a simple definition. It is generally accepted however, that staff development refers to the process whereby employees of an organisation enhance their knowledge and skills in directions that are advantageous to their role in the organisation. Definitions of staff development may be approached from the perspectives of the developer, the employer and the person being developed. O'Leary (1997) argued that staff development activity has to be outcome and process orientated, while Collett and Davidson (1997) suggested that a significant component of staff development is to facilitate change on a personal, professional and institutional level. Webb (1996) highlighted the need for human understanding and recognition that the feelings, emotions, humanity and 'being' of the people involved play an important part in staff development. This 'being' of the people was reinforced by Thornton and McEntee (1998) who viewed staff development as self development guided by critical questions and practised within frameworks that can lead to meeting the needs of all persons involved in the process. Essentially, staff development is an on-going process of education, training, learning and support activities and is concerned with helping people to grow within the organisations in which they are employed. An emphasis on lifelong learning, personal growth and fulfilment underlines the importance of sustained development. While the term 'staff development' has been defined in a number of ways, the primary purpose of academic staff development is to expand the educators' awareness of the various tasks they must undertake to contribute to the effective education of their students and the accomplishment of the organisation's objectives. Broadly, these tasks will include those associated with teaching and learning, research and scholarship, professional updating, administration and management. For most educators, learning and teaching activities will be central and staff development will include an in-depth consideration of learning and teaching situations so the educators are able to adjust and develop their teaching competencies and activities.

- The contemporary Higher Education (HE) culture of quality and audit places demands on healthcare educators for sustained high quality of teaching, for keeping up to date professionally, for effective administrative procedures and for research and scholarship.
- Work-based learning needs to be at the heart of staff development. Real life situations provide a focus for the process of reflection and the development and maintenance of skills.
- Particular challenges for new lecturers include the need to perform in the roles of scholar/researcher and teacher.
- In HE, careers may be characterised by different combinations involving teaching, research and management.

DISCUSSION

The cultural context of staff development

Institutional culture is characterised by the complex set of values and beliefs of the institution's staff. An enabling culture, in terms of staff development, is one that values individuals and gives the highest priority to professional development in order to transform professional practice and enhance job satisfaction.

External agencies influence culture by exercising indirect control over institutions, with increasing levels of accountability required for teaching and research. Best practice is identified and sustained through quality assurance and enhancement. The challenges, opportunities and issues for staff development are mainly a response to these initiatives. For example, in the United Kingdom (UK), a review of care in the National Health Service recommended that the maintenance of quality at the heart of patient care and service delivery required the healthcare educators to keep up to date, encourage staff development and accept responsibility for change (Darzi, 2008).

There are numerous frameworks and approaches to staff development including Investors in People (IIP) (2004), the European Foundation for Quality Management (EFQM) (2003) and the UK's Higher Education Academy (2004). These systems, techniques and strategies have a strong focus on the professional development of all academic staff. Teaching and research are, in principle, equally important in HE, with research, reflection and enquiry being essential tools in the development of educators able to interrogate the production and communication of knowledge in their discipline.

Developing and maintaining the skills of educators in healthcare

Sound academic development, involving research, scholarship and pedagogy, is necessary to move healthcare education forward. The challenges for the

key concepts in
healthcare education

educators include the need to keep abreast of a range of curricular and policy imperatives, as well as acquiring the skills to respond to the needs of students.

At an individual level, educators can be helped to identify their development needs in a number of ways, including self review, job analysis, peer review, informal discussion with their line manager or an individual appraisal interview.

Development can be enabled through observation, reflection, planning and action. Critical to the success of these approaches is the need for flexibility when engaging with the process rather than a mechanical routine approach. Individuals can learn alone or in a collaborative context and contributions from co-participants can encourage and make professional development more likely. Lifelong learning is central to developing and maintaining skills. Watson and Harris (1999) described the process as one that never formally starts or ends and viewed lifelong learning as an on-going process of critical reflection and questioning to arrive at new information or knowledge to inform action. Weick (1995) considered lifelong learning as a sense-making process of constructing, filtering, framing and creating. Clearly, for effective staff development, it is necessary to work flexibly and eclectically in order to meet the demands of each situation. Reliance on any one approach may hinder effective development.

Challenges for new educators

It is important to recognise that new educators in HE have their own distinctive development needs. Trowler and Knight (1999) discussed the socialisation of new entrants to HE and recognised how crucial the development process is. New educators need to be enabled to deal with the fundamentals of developing their teaching and research. They must also become engaged in academic communication structures, committees, quality assurance processes and curriculum development to meet new agendas. Central to self development is self-directed learning, with the individual having the opportunity to control aspects of their learning and construct meaningful learning experiences that enable improvements in knowledge and competency. The development of professional competence involves the acquisition of skills and ability, evidenced through performance tasks. As educators become reflectively aware of the behaviour, attitudes and motivations manifested in their performances, they are able to control the sort of person they want to become as educators.

Personal factors play a part in the individual's stance in relation to the development process; each person will have his or her own learning style and the way that the individual strives to achieve meaning in the learning process is an important consideration in the management of the staff development process.

Career pathways

As careers develop they reflect and influence personal development and can be facilitated by a variety of processes, role models and forms of mentorship.

Engagement in staff/self development should be seen as an excellent invest-ment for moving towards career goals. Staff who seek opportunities and adapt to change should achieve direct career-related benefits.

CASE STUDY

Susan is a senior lecturer in her second year of employment in HE. She had a good performance record, her specialism was paediatric nursing and she taught on the pre-registration nurse education programme. In her annual staff development interview Susan reviewed her work activities against her job description and outlined her staff development experiences since the last review. She wanted to enhance her skills in research and clinical practice and agreed a clinical development opportunity with her line manager.

Susan made contact with a senior manager in her link area and identified a small-scale research project to review the achievements and behavioural changes of qualified staff following the successful completion of an educa-tional programme in paediatric intensive care nursing. Susan was given time remission to lead the project. The outcomes were a 15,000 word research report, a paper presentation at a national conference and a publication in a refereed journal.

Susan's self direction and determination to meet her development needs were rewarded by this successful development experience. She had enhanced her research skills and partnership working. It is recognised by Turner and Harkin (2003) that self-directed professional development is likely to have a more sustained impact than development in which the educators are coerced to participate. Susan's approach to her staff development created an oppor-tunity for HE and clinical service to work collaboratively and explore educa-tion, clinical practice and clinical staff development. Susan felt valued in being given this learning opportunity and, due to her planning and organisa-tion, the project succeeded and impacted positively on her learning and teaching.

CONCLUSION

Staff development is both complex and straightforward. It is complex in the number of interpretations, perspectives and processes that can be entailed. It is straightforward in its focus on the development of individuals in ways that suit them and their organisations. Effective staff development is characterised by two components: the individual's professional development and the organisational development process. The two combine in a partnership for staff development. An effective staff development process is supportive of the individual and beneficial for the organisation. The developer helps the indi-vidual identify learning needs, the individual advises on the input and goals that are required. The organisation invests in the individual and the developed individual benefits the organisation. In an effective process the individual feels valued and develops confidence, and the organisation receives an enhanced input from the individual. Different visions will inform the process. Educators in HE may see themselves as teachers, as researchers, as managers or, primarily, as professionals. An effective developer provides a framework for educators and uses their expertise to help them to develop their career aspirations through learning projects that enable the educators' self determination to achieve their career goals.

It is truly the role of HE institutions to invest in the development of their people. Thus the success of the institution and the fulfilment of its staff are assured.

See also: experiential and work-based learning; interprofessional learning; leadership and management in academia; learning styles; peer support and observation; quality assurance and enhancement; reflection; research and scholarly activity

FURTHER READING

Barnett, R. (2005) *Reshaping the University: New Relationships between Research, Scholarship and Teaching.* Maidenhead: Open University Press.

REFERENCES

Collett, P. and Davidson, M. (1997) 'Re-negotiating autonomy and accountability: the professional growth of developers in a South African institution', *International Journal for Academic Development*, 2 (2): 28–34.

Darzi, A. (2008) *High Quality Care for All, NHS Next Stage Review. Final Report.* London: Department of Health.

European Foundation for Quality Management (2003) *EFQM Annual Report 2003.* Brussels: European Foundation for Quality Management.

Higher Education Academy (2004) *The UK Professional Standards Framework for Teaching and Supporting Learning in Higher Education.* York: HEA.

Investors in People (2004) Retrieved from Investors in People website: www.iipuk.co.uk/TheStandard/default.htm

O'Leary, J. (1997) 'Staff development in a climate of economic rationalism: a profile of the academic staff developer', *International Journal for Academic Development*, 2 (2): 72–82.

Thornton, L.J. and McEntee, M.E. (1998) 'Staff development as self development: extension and application of Russo's humanistic-critical theory approach for humanistic education and social action integration', *Humanistic Education and Development*, 36 (3): 143–59.

Trowler, P. and Knight, P.T. (1999) 'Organisational socialisation and induction in universities: reconceptualising theory and practice', *Higher Education*, 37 (2): 177–95.

Turner, G. and Harkin, J. (2003) *Factors Involved in the Facilitation of the Self-directed Professional Development of Teachers.* Loughborough: National Association of Staff Development.

Watson, T. and Harris, P. (1999) *The Emergent Manager.* London: Sage.

Webb, G. (1996) *Understanding Staff Development.* Buckingham: Open University Press.

Weick, K.E. (1995) *Sense Making in Organisations.* London: Sage.

2 assessment

Janice Gidman with case study by Janine Upton

DEFINITION

The dictionary definition of assessment is 'to evaluate or estimate' (Oxford English Dictionary, 2009). Assessment has a range of functions, including motivating students, identifying strengths and weaknesses, monitoring progress, confirming the achievement of learning objectives, providing feedback, judging competence and evaluating the effectiveness of teaching (Allin and Turnock, 2007). The purpose of assessment can be formative or summative. Formative assessment mainly focuses on assessment to promote on-going learning, whereas summative assessment focuses on verification that the student meets the requirements either to progress to the next level or to achieve an academic and/ or professional award. Boud and Falchikov (2006) also state that assessment should have a long-term emphasis on promoting continuing, lifelong learning in addition to the short-term focus of the specific education programme.

The timing of assessment can be continuous or episodic. Continuous assessment refers to the on-going assessment of learning, either formally or informally, throughout a programme of study, which focuses on assessment *for* learning (formative) as a key strategy to promote development. Episodic assessment occurs at set points during the programme and tends to focus on assessment *of* learning (summative), making a judgement on students' progress towards pre-determined outcomes of learning. The measurement of assessment can be norm referenced or criterion referenced. Norm referencing involves judging a student's performance against that of other students at the same stage of the programme, whereas criterion referencing entails judgements against objective outcomes. It is evident that norm referencing can lead to subjectivity and potential bias in assessment, particularly when considered in the context of practice assessment that involves a diverse group of practitioner assessors. The objectivity of assessment involves consideration of validity, reliability and practicality of the strategies selected.

KEY POINTS

- Assessment is an integral part of the learning process.
- Assessment should be *for* and *of* learning and should promote lifelong development.

- Assessment should be constructively aligned with learning outcomes, content and teaching strategies.
- Lecturers and practitioners need to use a range of strategies to assess competence within professional programmes.

DISCUSSION

Professional education occurs in the context of multiple interests, including professional bodies, government, employers and service users. This means that students undertaking these programmes are subject to a number of competing agendas, including prescribed curricula content, developing skills for learning, critical thinking, promoting conceptual understanding and connecting areas of theory and practice (Eraut, 2005). This is particularly relevant to curricula that prepare health professionals for registration. Students undertaking these programmes complete a range of practice placements and are assessed in both the theoretical and practical aspects of the programmes. The extensive literature related to professional education highlights the need for practitioners to be fit for practice at the point of qualification, maintaining the interests of public safety, whilst adopting the ethos of higher education to empower students throughout their studies (Stark and Stronach, 2006). However, the tensions within professional education are evident, in terms of the nature of knowledge in theory and practice and the professional regulatory body requirements to achieve prescribed competencies at the point of qualification (Cowan et al., 2005). It is apparent, therefore, that students undertaking professional programmes need to develop competence in its broadest sense, including personal and professional development. Contemporary definitions of competence incorporate cognitive, behavioural and affective dimensions and require practitioners, in both academic and practice settings, to have the knowledge and skills to use a range of assessment strategies.

Effective assessment

Assessment is a complex process. It has to do 'double-duty' (Boud, 2000) in that it needs to encompass formative assessment *for* learning and summative certification *of* learning; focus on the immediate task and promote continued learning and attend to both the process and content of learning. In addition, professional programmes have to meet the expectations of multiple stakeholders, including students, lecturers, the university, employers, government and professional regulatory bodies. In the United Kingdom (UK), the Quality Assurance Agency (QAA) (2006) has recognised the tensions inherent in the assessment process and has published a comprehensive guide for educators to promote the integration of assessment *of* learning and assessment *for* learning. Assessment is at the heart of the learning process for students (James et al., 2002) and Table 2.1 outlines 12 principles to ensure that assessment is effective.

It is a particular challenge to ensure the quality of assessment within practice settings, due to the diversity of organisations and the large number of

Table 2.1 Twelve principles of effective assessment

1 Assessment should help students to learn
2 Assessment must be consistent with the programme outcomes and content (constructive alignment)
3 Using a range of assessment strategies ensures that all aspects of competence are assessed and keeps students interested
4 Students need to clearly understand what is expected of them
5 Assessment criteria need to be detailed, transparent and justifiable
6 Students need specific, constructive and timely feedback following assessment
7 Overassessment may be counter-productive
8 Assessors need to be able to justify their decisions
9 Careful design of assessment tasks discourages plagiarism
10 Group assessment needs careful planning and detailed structure
11 It is important to ensure that assessment tasks are relevant to the diverse student group
12 It is important to critically evaluate the effectiveness of assessment in the curriculum

Source: Adapted from James et al., 2002

individuals involved. The complexity of assessment within the clinical practice area has long been recognised in the literature, with particular challenges in relation to the validity and reliability of assessment tools (Chambers, 1998). Additionally, it has been argued that, in recent years, theory and practice have been separated and that it is essential to integrate these within professional programmes (Maben et al., 2006). It follows, therefore, that assessment of professional knowledge and skills should not be artificially split into theoretical and practice assessment. Consequently, effective assessment within professional programmes requires a partnership approach between the university and the practitioners who are responsible for students' learning in practice settings.

Assessment strategies

There is a wide range of strategies available for lecturers and practitioners (summarised in Table 2.2) and a combination of these is essential to assess all aspects of competence.

The UK Centre for Legal Education (2008) advises lecturers to adopt innovative assessment strategies to meet the full range of students' learning styles, to broaden their approaches to learning and to ensure that assessment is integrated and relevant to the programme. For example, they contend that self-assessment and reflective accounts promote self-awareness, reflection and personal development. Portfolios incorporate these assessment strategies and they have become increasingly popular within higher education programmes to support development for both students and lecturers (Baume, 2003). Portfolios provide the opportunity for students to gather and present a wide range of evidence and to demonstrate achievement of professional competence, which is supported by a critical, reflective commentary. Portfolios are based on experiential learning theory, recognising that experience

Table 2.2 Strategies for the assessment of professional competence

Assessment strategies	
Multiple choice examinations	Reflection
Open question examinations	Journals
Tests	Portfolios
Assignments	Critical incident analysis
Case studies	Self assessment
Scenarios	Peer assessment
Seminar presentations	Service user assessment
Questioning	

alone is not sufficient for learning. Rather, students need to reflect on their experience; to conceptualise new rules for action and to test those rules in future situations (Webb, 2008).

CASE STUDY

The Diversity of Care module sits in the third trimester of the second year of a pre-qualifying nursing studies programme. The aim of the module is to offer students the opportunity to negotiate and explore a range of experiences, in traditional and non-traditional settings, potentially anywhere in the world. The module enables students to reflect on the impact of the 'diversity of care' experience in relation to their personal philosophy of care. Understandably, the diversity module is very popular with the students.

The module team were keen to ensure that the assessment for the module was constructively aligned with the learning outcomes and content. The assessment, therefore, consisted of an assignment reflecting on the achievement of the individual's negotiated practice outcomes and a presentation to peers. This ensured that the academic level of the student's work could be assessed by lecturers and also provided an opportunity for peer assessment by colleagues. The module team consider that the whole assessment process contributes to student learning. However, it is clear that the assignment provides the opportunity for the assessment *of* learning (against specified, measurable outcomes) and the presentation promotes the assessment *for* learning (providing an opportunity for discussion and critical reflection on each student's experience and personal philosophy of care).

CONCLUSION

It is evident from the above discussion that assessment is integral to the learning process and that this should include assessment *for* learning as well as assessment *of* learning. Programme development needs to ensure that assessment strategies are constructively aligned with learning outcomes, content and teaching strategies. It is also apparent that assessment within professional education programmes is complex and that it requires lecturers and practitioners to have the knowledge and skills to apply a range of strategies to assess competence.

See also: curriculum models and design; dealing with failing and problem students; feedback and marking; mentorship; practice teaching; service user and carer involvement; simulated learning and OSCEs; specific learning needs of students

FURTHER READING

Mullholland, J. and Turnock, C. (2000) *Learning in the Workplace: A Tool Kit for Placement Tutors, Supervisors, Mentors and Facilitators; Assessment in Practice*. Retrieved from Making Practice-based Learning Work website: www.practicebasedlearning.org/resources/assessment/intro.htm

Quality Assurance Agency for Higher Education (2007) *Integrative Assessment: Balancing Assessment of and Assessment for Learning*. Retrieved from the QAA website: www.enhancementthemes.ac.uk/themes/IntegrativeAssessment/IABalancing.asp

REFERENCES

Allin, L. and Turnock, C. (2007) *Assessing Student Performance in Work-based Learning*. Retrieved from Making Practice-based Learning Work website: www.practicebasedlearning.org/resources/materials/docs/Assessment%20in%20the%20Work%20Place/index.htm

Baume, D. (2003) *Supporting Portfolio Development*. Retrieved from HEA website: www.heacademy.ac.uk/assets/York/documents/resources/resourcedatabase/id295Supporting_Portfolio_Development.pdf

Boud, D. (2000) 'Sustainable assessment: rethinking assessment for the learning society', *Studies in Continuing Education*, 22 (2): 151–67.

Boud, D. and Falchikov, N. (2006) 'Aligning assessment with long term learning', *Assessment and Evaluation in Higher Education*, 31 (4): 399–413.

Chambers, M.A. (1998) 'Some issues in the assessment of clinical practice: a review of the literature', *Journal of Clinical Nursing*, 7: 201–8.

Cowan, D.T., Norman, I. and Coopamah, V.P. (2005) 'Competence in nursing practice: a focused review of literature', *Nurse Education Today*, 25 (5): 355–62.

Eraut, M. (2005) 'Continuity of learning', *Learning in Health and Social Care*, 4 (1): 1–6.

James, R., McInnis, C. and Devlin, M. (2002) *Getting Started with Student Assessment. Basic Advice for People New to University Teaching*. Retrieved from the Centre for the Study of Higher Education: Assessing Learning in Australian Universities website: www.cshe.unimelb.edu.au/assessinglearning/docs/Group.pdf

Maben, J., Latter, S. and MacLeod Clark, J. (2006) 'The theory–practice gap: impact of professional-bureaucratic work conflict on newly-qualified nurses', *Journal of Advanced Nursing*, 55 (4): 465–77.

Oxford English Dictionary (2009) Retrieved from OED website: www.askoxford.com

Stark, S. and Stronach, I. (2006) 'Nursing policy paradoxes and educational implications', in T. Warne and S. McAndrew (eds), *Using Patient Experience in Nurse Education*. Basingstoke: Palgrave Macmillan.

Quality Assurance Agency for Higher Education (2006) *Code of Practice: Section 6 Assessment of Students*. Retrieved from QAA website: www.qaa.ac.uk/academicinfrastructure/codeOfPractice/section6/COP_AOS.pdf

UK Centre for Legal Education (2008) *Assessment for Learning: A Guide for Law Teachers.* Retrieved from UKCLE website: www.ukcle.ac.uk/resources/assessment/guide/index. html

Webb, J. (2008) *Portfolio Based Learning and Assessment.* Retrieved from UKCLE website: www.ukcle.ac.uk/resources/trns/portfolios/index.html

3 behavioural learning theories

Andrew Lovell

DEFINITION

Behavioural learning theory outlines a model of how people learn from their experience, much of our behavioural responses being conditioned by events from our background and early experience. We learn from our daily experience, encounters of new situations, responding in the ways we think best suit the occasion and accumulating knowledge of the likely consequences to our behaviour. We also learn directly from formal learning situations.

> Behaviourism is a theory of learning focusing on observable behaviours and discounting any mental activity. Learning is defined simply as the acquisition of new behaviour. (Pritchard, 2005: 7)

KEY POINTS

- Behaviour that is followed by a reinforcing consequence will continue or strengthen.
- Behaviour that is followed by a punishing consequence will decrease or weaken.
- Behaviour that is not reinforced will not continue, it will gradually cease to occur or be extinguished.
- Reinforcers and punishers are defined by the effect they have on behaviour, rather than a particular judgement as to the degree of unpleasantness or whether they are aversive.

behavioural learning theories

11

- Negative reinforcement does not mean punishment but refers to a stimulus that, if removed upon a certain response, results in an increase in the probability of that response in similar future circumstances.

DISCUSSION

The emergence of behaviourism

The emphasis on the objective measurement of observable behaviour, as a means of psychological investigation, emerged at the beginning of the twentieth century, replacing introspection, the previously dominant method (Stapleton, 2001). 'Classical conditioning' refers to the process by which an association is made from an experience and subsequent learning takes place; the success or failure that a student, for example, associates with a given learning situation will govern future behaviour. The term 'behaviourism' is associated with Watson (1913), but the emergent behavioural approach is most associated with Thorndike (1931), specifically the 'law of effect', wherein a cat comes to learn that by pressing a bar it will receive food. Pavlov (1927) used dogs to demonstrate the principle of 'extinction', whereby the sound of a bell meant the appearance of food and induced salivation, but ceased to have any meaning if the food failed to appear, salivation thus disappearing. These early experiments led to the concept of Stimulus–Response (S–R) learning, consisting of the acquisition of skills or responses as a consequence of environmental manipulation and behaviours subsequently eliminated, increased, decreased and generalised (Ashman and Conway, 1997). The key shift, of course, was the later application of behavioural principles to human subjects, seemingly simple but extremely powerful in shaping learning, both in practice and education.

These early principles thus paved the way for the emergence of 'operant conditioning', which is based on sequences of learning in which each new step is dependent upon those previously acquired. The selection of the learning step arises from the task analysis, breaking the skill into a precise sequence of logical events in order to achieve the goal. Skinner (1953, 1971), over several decades, was hugely significant in the consolidation of behavioural theory and the elaboration of its key principles. 'Shaping' relates to the reward of successive approximations prior to a behaviour being learned, and 'generalisation' refers to the application of a behaviour to other circumstances, the construction of an assignment, for example, providing the requisite skills for many other forms of project work.

A model for understanding behaviour

At the heart of behavioural learning theory lies the antecedent–behaviour–consequence framework (A–B–C model), the dismantling of a learning situation into its critical component parts (see Table 3.1).

Antecedents and consequences comprise events influencing behaviour, both environmental, such as the telephone ringing, or internal sensations, like

Table 3.1 The A–B–C model

Antecedent	Behaviour	Consequence
A stimulus that acts as a the trigger for the current behaviour	What the person does and says	A stimulus that provides the motivation to behave in a similar or different way on the next occasion

Source: Adapted from McBrien and Felce, 2000

pain or hunger. The model goes some way to explaining human behaviour by contextualizing it, providing the circumstances within which it occurs and the subsequent likelihood of a person reacting in a similar way on subsequent occasions. The antecedent column will contain information such as the date of submission for an assignment. The subsequent behaviour surrounds the construction of the assignment of requisite length and as an accurate response to the assignment brief, whilst the resultant pass should provide motivation as to the submission of the next assignment. Consequences likely to strengthen the association between the situation and a response act as 'reinforcers', and those that weaken the association serve as 'punishers'. Table 3.2 identifies different forms of reinforcement and punishment.

Positive reinforcement refers to when a rewarding consequence occurs as a result of the behaviour, thus increasing the likelihood of its recurring in similar circumstances. Negative reinforcement, however, relates to the way in which an unpleasant situation comes to an end as a consequence of the behaviour; the person becomes more likely to behave similarly in the future,

Table 3.2 Effects of different behavioural consequences

		Stimulus presented	Stimulus removed
N	R	**Positive reinforcement**	**Negative punishment**
A	E		
T	I	e.g. material reward, give compliment,	e.g. fine money, automatic fail for
U	N	financial remuneration, academic	plagiarism, academic penalty for
R	F	success	late submission
E	O		
	R		
O	C		
F	E	**Encourages behaviour**	**Discourages behaviour**
	R		
S	P	**Positive punishment**	**Negative reinforcement**
T	U		
I	N	e.g. direct criticism of academic	e.g. avoid difficult demand, avoid
M	I	work, exertion of pressure	formal presentation
U	S	to perform practical task	
L	H		
U	E		
S	R	**Discourages behaviour**	**Encourages behaviour**

Source: Adapted from McBrien and Felce, 2000

the reward having been the removal of something that they had not liked. Neither positive nor negative refer to good or bad in behavioural theory, rather they are technical descriptions of the ways in which behaviours are reinforced, the individual being motivated or encouraged to repeat their actions in similar circumstances. Unfortunately, as Sheldon points out, 'Negative reinforcement is a clumsy term and … causes students of learning theory more trouble than anything else' (1995: 63).

Punishment continues to cause debate and controversy, not least because of behaviourism's historical association with aversive interventions, particularly with vulnerable groups (Lovett, 1996). It is important, nevertheless, if only to understand the role that punishment has played in an individual's development. Behaviour is punished by the implementation of something unpleasant as a result of that behaviour (positive punishment) or if something desirable comes to an end as a consequence of the behaviour (negative punishment). A consistent pattern of punishment also causes learning, reducing the likelihood of particular behaviour continuing to occur. The person, effectively, learns not to engage in the behaviour, adjusting their reactions accordingly; the consistent lack of response to an assignment draft, for example, is likely to result in a student seeking support through some alternative means.

The critique of behavioural learning theory

Behavioural learning theory has been subject to considerable critique, the seemingly innocuous operation of the principle of reinforcement, for example, disguising its considerable power in changing behaviour. The early experimentation with animals to demonstrate the stimulus–response link presumes a similarly mechanistic relationship when applied to human beings. Some early research on learning situations, however, suggested that individuals often learn quite complex internal representations, which are not evident in their immediate actions but can be used to generate different behaviours according to the situation (Tolman, 1932). Initial learning might be explicable by linking together simple learning experiences, but later learning involves an overall perspective and the capacity to derive new ways of seeing by drawing on previous experience and knowledge (Long, 2006). The most effective critique of behavioural learning, therefore, concerns the role of underlying mental representations and abilities, the basis of the alternative broad approach to learning characterising the twentieth century, cognitive-interactionism. The behaviourally orientated educator tries to change the observable behaviours of students in a significant way, whereas the cognitive-interactionist seeks to help students develop their understandings of significant problems and situations (Bigge and Shermis, 1999).

CASE STUDY

Sharaz is a post-registration student who is working full-time as a community nurse with people with learning disabilities whilst he is studying part-time for his degree. He is a diligent individual with good organisational and time management skills, though he struggles with the complexity of following an individually tailored educational programme. Sharaz receives a half-day each week as study time, which he finds invaluable for attending the taught part of each module; he also has opportunity to arrange his working week in such a way as to accommodate attendance at tutorials and occasional visits to the library. His registration on the degree programme with the university enables him to access the institutional intranet, which contains useful information on the various learning and support services provided for students, as well as facilitating access to module resources, such as online articles and book chapters. Each of these elements – study time, work flexibility, tutorial time and online resources – provides Sharaz with positive reinforcement for pursuing his goal of a degree, something that he has sought since completing his diploma some 15 years ago.

Studying independently at degree level has not proved straightforward for Sharaz and he has occasionally encountered obstacles to his progress that have been difficult for him to overcome. An attempt to shorten the time it would take him to complete his degree by undertaking two modules simultaneously, for example, was met with a refusal by his line manager to grant Sharaz a full day of each week as study time. His manager determined that it was Sharaz's decision to commit to two modules and the Trust had no obligation to increase the support he was receiving. Furthermore, an attempt to request financial support, since each module was costing around £400, met with an immediate refusal, and ultimately meant that Sharaz had to withdraw from pursuing the two modules during the same semester because of the cost. Sharaz's subsequent meeting with his manager revealed that he was actually reluctant to support him in his studies at all, because he regarded the degree, a professional practice qualification, to be the wrong one. His line manager regarded the specialist practice degree to be the appropriate qualification, something that Sharaz had discussed at length with his previous line manager, who had ultimately supported his decision to complete his degree over a longer period because of family commitments and because he regarded the degree content to be most pertinent to his work. The lack of study time support, prohibitive financial burden and disagreement over the relevance of the qualification to his work all constituted negative punishment, potentially very damaging to both his working life and likelihood of educational success. Sharaz reacted by becoming less committed to the Trust and more determined to complete his degree. He found the expected presence of his line manager acted as negative reinforcement, wherein he would seek to leave a multi-disciplinary meeting or avoid attending. The A–B–C model informs us that this anticipated presence precipitates Sharaz's non-attendance resulting in an increasingly dysfunctional relationship.

CONCLUSION

The behavioural approach continues to make a serious contribution to the understanding of human learning, emphasising the specific context framing our experience, the power of reinforcement and the analysis of actions according to their component parts. The sometime aversive history of behaviourism urges us to seriously question the relationship between punishment and learning; it is evident, furthermore, that we cannot extract cognition from the process, but, nevertheless, the insights of Skinner (1953, 1971) and others remain fundamental to our understanding of learning.

See also: assessment; clinical competence; cognitive learning theories; curriculum models and design; humanist learning theories; practice teaching; simulated learning and OSCEs; teaching strategies

FURTHER READING

Salkind, N.J. (2004) *An Introduction to Theories of Human Development*. London: Sage.
Skinner, B.F. (1973) *Beyond Freedom and Dignity*. Harmondsworth: Penguin.

REFERENCES

Ashman, A.F. and Conway, R.N.F. (1997) *An Introduction to Cognitive Education: Theory and Applications*. London: Routledge.

Bigge, M.L. and Shermis, S.S. (1999) *Learning Theories for Teachers*. New York: Longman.

Long, M. (2006) *The Psychology of Education*. London: Routledge.

Lovett, H. (1996) *Learning to Listen: Positive Approaches and People with Difficult Behaviour*. London: Jessica Kingsley.

McBrien, J. and Felce, D. (2000) *Working with People who have Severe Learning Difficulty and Challenging Behaviour: A Practical Handbook on the Behavioural Approach*. Kidderminster: British Institute of Learning Disabilities.

Pavlov, I.P. (1927) *Conditional Reflexes*. London: Oxford University Press.

Pritchard, A. (2005) *Ways of Learning: Learning Theories and Learning Styles in the Classroom*. London: Fulton.

Sheldon, B. (1995) *Cognitive Behavioural Therapy: Research, Practice and Philosophy*. London: Routledge.

Skinner, B.F. (1953) *Science and Human Behaviour*. London: Collier Macmillan.

Skinner, B.F. (1971) *Beyond Freedom and Dignity*. New York: Alfred A. Knopf.

Stapleton, M. (2001) *Psychology in Practice: Education*. London: Hodder and Stoughton.

Thorndike, E.L. (1931) *Human Learning*. New York: Appleton–Century–Croft.

Tolman, E.C. (1932) *Purposive Behaviour in Animals and Men*. New York: Century.

Watson, J.B. (1913) 'Psychology as the behaviourist views it', *Psychological Review*, 20: 157–8.

4 clinical competence

Tracey Proctor-Childs

DEFINITION

The notion of competence, its definition, assessment and measurement are complex and clouded by the current political and professional debates about the delivery of care, workforce needs and the ever-changing fluctuations in service reorganisation (Murrells et al., 2009; Scholes, 2006). There is a significant amount of literature on the development of competence, however the definitions are varied and to an extent context-specific. Riitta-Liisa et al. (2008), in an extensive literature review of competence in intensive and critical care nursing, indentified four main domains of clinical and professional competence: skills acquisition; knowledge; attitudes and values; and experience. These are recurring themes in the literature (Flanagan et al., 2000; Kim, 2007; Lofmark et al., 1999; Manley and Garbett, 2000). The older literature now appears dated, as the idea of competence has become a familiar concept to healthcare educators, who are confident in determining how to set and achieve competences as part of curriculum development and delivery.

Eraut (1994), in considering competence from an educational perspective, recognises that competence is not an end-point but rather it is part of the development of expertise and is an intrinsic aspect of professional practice. There are thus several dimensions of competence, from undergraduate students (who need to practise safely and effectively at the point of registration), to those for whom competence reflects a highly complex and dynamic process of learning through experience (improving decision making, judgement and reflexivity). These opposite ends of the continuum meet the varied needs of practitioners at different stages of their professional development. Competence is concerned, therefore, not only with skills acquisition and application, but also with the development of knowledge to support decision making and assessment. This broad notion of competence also requires practitioners to understand accountability and ethical implications for practice in complex and fluid clinical situations.

KEY POINTS

- Contemporary perspectives of competence in healthcare are holistic, including knowledge, skills, values and ethics.
- Assessment of competence in healthcare programmes is a complex and demanding process.

- Failing to fail students is an area of current concern in professional programmes.
- Mentors and practice supervisors need preparation and support to assess the competence of healthcare students.

DISCUSSION

The rise in competence as a basis for professional care in the United Kingdom has been driven by the current political agendas for a more flexible, multi-professional workforce that can deliver the modernisation agenda and address the skills shortage in some key areas, for example critical care. If the starting point of competence is skills acquisition, it can be seen that this will enable a workforce who may not want or need to achieve professional registration to meet the requirements of a service in an effective and efficient manner. Whilst for some practitioners and educationalists this is profoundly uncomfortable, the recipient of care surely has a right to expect at the very least a practitioner (whether qualified or unqualified) who is competent in their sphere of practice. For qualified practitioners, research suggests that competence that has been assessed either by themselves or practice assessors gives a more confident and self reliant practitioner (Cowan et al., 2007; Kim, 2007).

Critiques of competence-based education approaches

The reductionist approach to the development of professional practice is something that has caused concern in an area that requires a level of holistic skills to practise competently (McMullan et al., 2003). It is evident that there are contradictions inherent between educational philosophy, which is mainly humanistic in its approach, and the behavioural objectives that are often used to assess professional performance. The emergence of measurable outcomes as indicators of the quality of education appears to be a politically, rather than an educationally, driven phenomenon. This may lead to a narrow, fragmented structure of education in which teaching is focused on examination and test results rather than on learning. The modular structure of many programmes is a good example of this – it may limit natural enquiry, devalue the affective domains in education and stifle the development of creative and innovative problem-solving in students. This includes communication and empathy, which although vital aspects of professional practice, are very difficult to write in terms of behavioural competences. However, competence also has many positive outcomes from a learner's perspective: it is transparent about what is to be learned, the progress of the learner can be demonstrated, and teaching and learning activities are constructed to ensure that learners meet the outcomes. A competence-based approach enables individual students' progress to be monitored and remedial action can be instigated if required. The outcomes also act as a positive re-enforcement for students who achieve outcomes quickly (Brady, 1996).

Assessing competence

Competence can be assessed in a variety of ways. The prerequisites for this are a clear and definable set of competences, so that learners and qualified practitioners are clear about what is to be judged, measured and assessed. It was noted above that competence is multi-dimensional, from a skilled level of performance that meets specific behavioural objectives (for example, dispensing medication to a patient) to a more complex skills set that includes expertise and the ability to work in complex and unpredictable situations. Attributable competence assessment considers individuals' characteristics and attempts to measure critical thinking skills, adaptability, problem-solving and self confidence in care delivery (Cassidy, 2009). The challenge for assessment of competence is to ensure that these polarities are addressed. As with any patient clinical assessment, consideration of the whole person (holism) can be transferred to the assessment process and integrate the interwoven knowledge, skills and attitudes necessary to deliver emotionally intelligent care. Norman et al. (2002) identify the difficulties in using valid and reliable methods to assess students' abilities and performance in care delivery activities, because of the paucity of research in using reliable measurement indicators for the assessment of competence.

The person on whom assessment of competence rests is the mentor or practice supervisor who makes the final decision about the achievement of professional competence. Whilst this may seem a straightforward role for registered practitioners it is in reality a complex process. The mentor/practice supervisor's primary method of assessment is through direct observation involving subjective judgements about a student's level of performance, knowledge and skills. The mentor/practice supervisor will have undergone a recognised period of training to develop the knowledge and skills required to 'sign off' the student as competent at the point of registration. He/she will also need to demonstrate professional values in carrying out the assessment. The clinical milieu in which mentors and practice supervisors work is a highly demanding arena, with a constant tension between clinical care, teaching and the learning needs of students. The assessment process may, therefore, become fragmented and this may inhibit the reliable assessment of students' competence (Manley and Garbett, 2000). A current concern, within healthcare programmes, is the inability of mentors to fail students who do not meet the required level of competence for safe and effective practice (Cassidy, 2009; Rutowski, 2007). This is an issue that all healthcare educators need to be aware of, as initiating the support mechanisms for mentors who fail students, as well as supporting students who fail, has assumed greater importance. There are many reasons suggested to explain this 'failure to fail'. These include concerns relating to lack of recognition that clinical assessment of competence is of equal value to the academic aspects of a student's journey, inadequate support for mentors and staff shortages. Perhaps the most concerning effect of this is the personal failure felt by mentors when failing a student.

They may feel that they could have provided a better learning environment or spent more time with the student, which leads to feelings of inadequacy and self doubt, resulting in mentors who are reluctant to supervise or fail future students (Dolan, 2003; Rutowski, 2007).

User involvement and developing self assessment of competence

The emphasis on competence has increased with the need to ensure that practitioners are skilled and safe to work with, and deliver care to, the public at a minimum standard. The assumption that, as part of patient and public involvement in care delivery, patients and service users wish to be equally involved in assessment of competence and can identify the skills and competence needed is one put forward by Norman et al. (2002). However, Calman (2006), in a study to explore this issue concludes that patients' ability to undertake this is influenced by the situation and choices available to refuse care. Service users were insightful in considering that one observation of performance of competence was not sufficient to judge the competence of that person overall.

Levett-Jones (2007), in considering the use of self assessment of competence, uses the vehicle of narrative to illuminate the clinical episode. For Levett-Jones this has facilitated the opportunity for nurses to explore the complexities of everyday practice and to reveal a new appreciation of clinical practice skills. This, for the students, led to a clear definition of their levels of competence in relation to those of a skilled registered practitioner. An essential aspect of professional development for students is to undertake structured facilitated reflection (Cowan et al., 2007; Kim, 2007) in order to examine their own practice and competence.

CASE STUDY

Becci is a staff nurse on a busy surgical ward. She has recently completed a mentor preparation programme and is currently supervising Jill, a third-year nursing student. Although Jill has excellent clinical skills, Becci is concerned about her interpersonal skills. Several patients have commented that Jill has been abrupt with them and discussion with colleagues confirmed these concerns. Becci has a very good relationship with Liz, the link lecturer for the ward, who was involved in her recent mentorship programme and who visits the ward regularly to support mentors. Becci raised her concerns with Liz and with the Practice Education Facilitator for the surgical directorate and they both encouraged her to discuss the issues with Jill. At the midpoint interview, Becci identified that Jill was still failing to achieve the expected outcomes for communication and a tripartite meeting was arranged to develop an action plan to address this. This example of effective partnership working ensured that Becci felt supported to address the issues with Jill and if she does not meet the communication outcomes by the end of her placement, it will be a joint decision that she fails.

CONCLUSION

In considering the complexities involved in defining competence it is evident that this is more complex than simple skills performance. Assessment of competence is both complex and demanding of both practitioners and educators but is a crucial part of professional accountability and responsibility. It is important for students to develop critical reflection skills alongside competence in order to continue to develop and enhance their professional development throughout their careers.

See also: assessment; behavioural learning theories; curriculum models and design; humanist learning theories; mentorship; practice teaching; reflection; service user and carer involvement

FURTHER READING

Eraut, M. (1994) *Developing Professional Knowledge and Competence.* London: The Falmer Press.
Scholes, J. (2006) *Developing Expertise in Critical Care Nursing.* Oxford: Blackwell.

REFERENCES

Brady, L. (1996) 'Outcome-based education: a critique', *The Curriculum Journal,* 7 (1): 5–16.

Calman, L. (2006) 'Patients' views of nurses' competence', *Nurse Education Today,* 26 (8): 719–25.

Cassidy, S. (2009) 'Interpretation of competence in student assessment', *Nursing Standard,* 23 (18): 39–46.

Cowan, D., Wilson-Barnett, J. and Norman, I. (2007) 'A European survey of general nurses' self assessment of competence', *Nurse Education Today,* 27 (5): 452–8.

Dolan, G. (2003) 'Assessing student nurses clinical competency: will we ever get it right?', *Journal of Clinical Nursing,* 12 (1): 132–41.

Eraut, M. (1994) *Developing Professional Knowledge and Competence.* London: The Falmer Press.

Flanagan, J., Baldwin, S. and Clarke, D. (2000) 'Work-based learning as a means of developing and assessing nursing competence', *Journal of Clinical Nursing,* 9 (3): 360–8.

Kim, K. (2007) 'Clinical competence among senior nursing students after their preceptorship experiences', *Journal of Professional Nursing,* 23 (6): 369–75.

Levett-Jones, T. (2007) 'Facilitating reflective practice and self assessment of competence through the use of narratives', *Nurse Education in Practice,* 7 (2): 112–19.

Lofmark, A., Hannersjo, S. and Wikblad, K. (1999) 'A summative evaluation of clinical competence: student and nurses perceptions of inpatients individual physical and emotional needs', *Journal of Advanced Nursing,* 9 (4): 942–9.

Manley, K. and Garbett, R. (2000) 'Paying Peter and Paul: reconciling concepts of expertise with competency for a clinical career structure', *Journal of Clinical Nursing,* 9 (3): 347–59.

McMullan, M., Endacott, R. and Gray, M.A. (2003) 'Portfolios and assessment of competence; a review of the literature', *Journal of Advanced Nursing,* 41 (3): 283–94.

Murrells, T., Robinson, S. and Griffiths, P. (2009) 'Assessing competence in nursing', *Nursing Management,* 16 (4): 18–19.

Norman, I., Watson, R., Murrells, T., Calman, L. and Redfern, S. (2002) 'The validity and reliability of methods to assess the competence to practice of pre-registration nursing and midwifery students', *International Journal of Nursing Studies,* 39 (2): 133–45.

Riitta-Liisa, A., Tarja, S. and Leino-Kilpi, H. (2008) 'Competence in intensive and critical care nursing: a literature review', *Intensive and Critical Care Nursing*, 24 (2): 78–89.

Rutkowski, K. (2007) 'Failure to fail: assessing nursing students' competence during practice placements', *Nursing Standard*, 22 (13): 35–40.

Scholes, J. (2006) *Developing Expertise in Critical Care Nursing*. Oxford: Blackwell.

5 cognitive learning theories

Mike Thomas

DEFINITION

Cognitive learning is considered to be an internal selected action involving a range of brain functions including thinking, perception, input, processing, memory and feelings (Gopee, 2008).

KEY POINTS

- Theories of cognitive learning include gestalt, schema (assimilation) and experiential learning.
- Cognitive learning theories (CLTs) arose out of a sense that behavioural learning theories were too constraining in their approaches to how learning occurred; they combine elements of behavioural and social learning theories.
- CLTs apply to health education and support problem-based curricula and methods of teaching such as experiential and participative learning.
- CLTs apply to healthcare practices with their approaches to new skills acquisition building upon previous experiences and assimilating into existing knowledge.

DISCUSSION

Cognitive learning theories arose out of the earlier pioneering work on learning carried out by the Behaviourist School. Proponents such as Pavlov, Watson,

Thorndyke and Skinner had established observable alterations in behaviour based on certain systems principles. Such alterations in behaviour were widely accepted as due learning processes. Pavlov was a Russian physiologist who gave the world *classical conditioning*, an important insight into anticipatory responses by the brain causing physiological alterations that would normally occur during a real event (Child, 1977). Watson, Thorndyke and Skinner worked in the United States of America. Watson founded the idea of connections (nowadays termed *behaviourism*) to describe a *stimulus–response* or trial and error connection to learning (a stimulus–response or S–R model) (Watson, 1931). Thorndyke, working contemporaneously, gave a similar model with his Laws of Effect which state that, in addition to S–R behaviour, the element of reward will reinforce certain behaviours whilst negative outcomes will decrease behavioural responses (Child, 1977). All three theorists, Pavlov, Watson and Thorndyke, demonstrated another effect: reinforcement must be regular and rewarding enough in repeated behaviour for effects to reoccur and be maintained. For example, it is not enough for a person to exercise or practise repeatedly for improvement to take place; the individual must know the results of the actions. Feedback, whether physiological or psychological, is important for behavioural change to occur.

Skinner (1953) coined the phrase *operant conditioning*. This described the phenomenon on trial and error learning leading to behaviour that is rewarded to the level whereby the behaviour is reinforced to a relatively fixed pattern or trait. The behaviour operates to fulfil a goal. Skinner developed the S–R model to such an extent that the nature, style and time frame of reward and subsequent behavioural patterns were refined. For example, in learning there should be small chunks of information rewarded with understanding (within the learner's capabilities) and feedback before further learning can occur. Behaviour can thus be changed in humans; for good or bad.

All these behaviourists gave great credence to experimental designs and measurable, observable behaviours. They were relatively uninterested in how the individual's perception of a situation may also serve a function in stimulus response. Cognitive theorists were, however, very interested in this area and argued that breaking down behavioural responses to connecting bits and pieces may camouflage the meaning of the behaviour itself to the individual. Kohler (1925), one of the originators of the Gestalt School, identified that putting a hungry rat or pigeon in a box full of levers and switches will in itself stimulate trial and error learning.

Brewer (1972) also highlighted the fact that human beings can differentiate internally between classical *reflex responses* (e.g. blinking or sneezing) and *operant responses* where the individual may just as likely respond based on what they think the person directing them wants to see. Groome (1999) summarised the cognitivist position by defining cognitive approaches as the way in which the brain processes information and how it takes in information, makes sense of it, and then uses the information to respond. Processes involve perception, memory storage and retrieval (recall), making choices and analysing the results of such choices.

Unlike behaviourists who examined defined separate but linked elements, classical, S–R and operant models; the *cognitivists* tend to see processes as intertwining and inseparable and therefore more difficult to present as separate entities. Perception, for example, is difficult to isolate from memory; recall from *reinforcers*, assimilation of new information from early learning experiences. Wertheimer (1945) and Kohler (1925), and Koffka (1935) gave us the Gestalt School (*gestalt* means 'shape'), and professed that individuals add information to what is perceived and often respond by selecting the most likely solution available at the time. Individuals can therefore confer a meaning to a situation before action occurs.

Bartlett (1932) proposed a different cognitive theory – the *Schema Model*. He suggested that new perceptions are compared with information already held in the memory and the individual therefore provides a rationale to situations which is adapted to past experiences and knowledge. Because everyone has different experiences and knowledge they will often perceive situations in different ways and react accordingly, an important consideration when teaching groups. Schematic approaches involve clustering groups of information around existing knowledge to build up a framework or structure to respond to the world. Both Gestalt and Schema learning are important with regards to the area of learning through insight. Work that involves problem-solving and feedback such as group seminars or supervision are particularly successful methods to support insight.

Tolman (1949) provided a further view of cognitive theory by proposing that learning itself is a goal-directed activity. Cues or signs are used to generate a pattern that makes goal attainment faster or easier. Rats, pigeons, dogs, chimpanzees or humans involved in behaviourist experiments did not therefore just connect or associate specific responses to stimuli. They instead assimilated cognitive meanings (sometimes referred to as cognitive maps) in order to develop and acquire patterns of responses. Ausubel et al. (1978) argued that meaningful learning occurs when new learning interacts with the knowledge already possessed by the individual. This is an important point because it explains the concept of *transferable skills*. For example, if a student is taught an assessment skill in a hospital setting they will also be able to assimilate the learning and adapt the skill in different settings such as a person's home. Ausubel et al.'s (1978) approach to assimilation also goes some way to support retention of knowledge that is increased if information is presented by the educationalist in a way that activates existing knowledge to demonstrate the link or meaning to the new learning about to take place.

Ausubel et al. (1978) distinguished between different types of learning approaches based on Tolman's early work. For example, giving too much knowledge in unrelated chunks does not increase learning. Educational approaches should therefore be based on meaningful learning whereby information is presented in a way that builds on earlier work and is represented to the learner in a context that provides meaning to them. In this way, a large body of knowledge can be assimilated in a relatively short space of time.

Discovery learning takes longer and incorporates guidance from a facilitator, so group work, seminars and individual supervision are good approaches to allow meaning and insight to be assimilated in a more exploratory way. Alternatively *rote learning* is useful only in the early stages of cognitive development such as infancy and childhood; it has little impact for adult learning as it has little interaction with past information and belittles the learning approach. An example would be asking a student to learn by rote the chambers of the heart or five pages from the British National Formula with no application of the knowledge of physiology/anatomy or pharmacology in a health context. Ausubel et al. (1978) stressed that the most important elements of teaching and learning are the interactions between the presented information and what the student already knows.

The assimilation of new knowledge into an existing cognitive framework builds a more detailed schematic structure. Discovering what the student already knows is therefore an important aspect of teaching. *Assimilation theory* is also used as a basis for a learning strategy known as advanced organiser. Ausubel and his colleagues present learning as more facilitative if the student is given material prior to the presentation of new knowledge (Ausubel et al., 1978). Prior reading, directing activities such as practice visits, e-pages for discussion on upcoming learning or a presentation at commencement of a lecture outlining aims, outcomes and content allow students to better assimilate the new information into existing schema when it is then presented.

Kolb (1984) advocated another cognitive approach; learning by doing rather than being informed by others. *Experiential learning* is now widely used within reflective models of learning and involves undertaking the experience, thinking about the experience (either during or after the event), exploring the impact on existing experiences and knowledge; generalising the learning gained from the experience and applying new learning in future situations. Such an approach to cognitive learning underpins the problem-based curriculum with its emphasis on portfolio learning, skills-based assessments, feedback and critical incidents seminars. Phillips et al. (2000) concluded that experiential reflective methods would be a stronger approach to knowledge acquisition using critical incident feedback sessions in mentoring, while Stuart (2007) looked at the work of several studies to conclude that combined methods of assessment are preferable to single approaches. This offered the most comprehensive meaning of the learning being taught and also prevented students focusing only on what they perceive to be important to the lecturer, rather than to themselves. A mix of lectures, discovery, self-directed and experiential learning with assessments such as observations, questioning, discussion, simulation, case presentation, portfolios, refection and assignments allow the most comprehensive approaches to enable learners to assimilate new learning into their existing knowledge. These also support motivation, personalities, group interaction and students' responses to the characteristics of the teacher (Quinn and Hughes, 2007).

CASE STUDY

Peter is a second-year mental health student about to commence his first placement in a forensic unit. He approaches his personal tutor, Jenny, to say that he has received no prior teaching sessions regarding forensic mental health and he is the only member of the cohort on the placement. He is anxious about his knowledge base, what the experience may entail and he feels a bit lonely without his fellow students there too.

Jenny listened to Peter and together they compiled a list of his main concerns in priority order. Top of the list was Peter's lack of knowledge regarding forensic care. Jenny provided Peter with a short reading list regarding forensic care and ensured she met him again in a week to spend time with him going through the articles and highlighting areas of knowledge that Peter already held. Jenny also introduced Peter to the link tutor for that placement who was able to see Peter fortnightly on the unit.

Peter was encouraged to contact the placement staff and arrange visits to the unit beforehand and discuss his preliminary perceptions with Jenny. The year tutor also contacted Peter to ensure that he participated in the online discussion board with his fellow students. On access, Peter discovered that the discussion area included a reflective group file which focused on learning events using a reflective model.

Three weeks into this placement Peter mentioned to his link tutor that the prior reading and discussions with Jenny, a pre-placement visit and the ongoing discussion board had given him confidence and allayed his anxieties. He continued to a successful completion of the placement.

CONCLUSION

Cognitive learning theories play an important part for educators in healthcare. The incorporation of early behaviourism with its emphasis on observable alterations in behaviour into a model that explored how behaviour altered has influenced education delivery in a substantial way. The emergence of problem-based curricula, experiential learning, reflection and different assessment approaches can be traced to cognitive theories around gestalt, schema, reward, assimilation and motivation. It is perhaps fitting to end with a view from Ausubel et al. (1978), which best summarises the cognitive learning approach; they opined that greater learning will take place when one finds out what it is that the student knows and takes this into account when selecting and applying the teaching style.

See also: behavioural learning theories; learning styles; teaching strategies; teaching styles

FURTHER READING

Bigge, M.L. and Shermis, S.S. (2004) *Learning Theories for Teachers*. Boston, MA: Pearson/ Allyn and Bacon.

REFERENCES

Ausubel, D., Novak, J. and Hanesian, H. (1978) *Educational Psychology – A Cognitive View*. New York: Holt, Rinehart and Winston.

Bartlett, F.C. (1932) *Remembering*. Cambridge: Cambridge University Press.

Brewer, W.F. (1972) *Cognitive and the Symbolic Processes*. University Park, PA: Pennsylvania State University.

Child, D. (1977) *Psychology and the Teacher*. London: Holt, Rinehart and Winston.

Groome, D. (1999) *An Introduction to Cognitive Psychology – Processes and Disorders*. East Sussex: Psychology Press Ltd.

Gopee, N. (2008) *Mentoring and Supervision in Healthcare*. London: Sage.

Koffka, K. (1935) *Principles of Gestalt Psychology*. New York: Harcourt Brace.

Kohler, W. (1925) *The Mentality of Apes*. New York: Harcourt Brace.

Kolb, D. (1984) *Experiential Learning: Experience as a Source of Learning and Development*. London: Prentice–Hall.

Phillips, T., Schostak, J. and Tyler, J. (2000) *Practice and Assessment in Nursing and Midwifery: Doing It for Real*. London: ENB.

Quinn, F.M. and Hughes, J.S. (2007) *Quinn's Principles and Practice of Nurse Education*, 5th edn. Cheltenham: Nelson Thornes.

Skinner, B.F. (1953) *Science and Human Behaviour*. New York: Macmillan.

Stuart, C.C. (2007) *Assessment, Supervision and Support in Clinical Practice*. Philadelphia: Churchill Livingstone Elsevier.

Tolman, E.C. (1949) *Purposive Behaviour in Animals and Men*. New York: Appleton–Century–Croft.

Watson, J.B. (1931) *Behaviourism*. New York: Routledge and Kegan Paul.

Wertheimer, M. (1945) *Productive Thinking*. New York: Harpo.

6 complexity theory

Helen Cooper

DEFINITION

Historically, the development of healthcare education reflects that of adult education. It can be traced from 'content-driven' through 'objectives-driven' and 'process-driven' (Ross, 2000), to research-led educational development (Brew, 2001). Given this focus, there is an increasing need for a theoretical framework that addresses its complex nature given that education is a continuous process that aims to promote connectivity between formal and informal learning. Much of learning is therefore emergent and, as educators, we are essentially engaged in a dynamic system, one that views learners' needs as heterogeneous and in a constant state of change. These ideas have much in common with a Complexity perspective.

In the context of Complexity there is no single unified theory, but several theories that have amalgamated from a range of natural sciences studying complex phenomena (e.g. physics, computer science, biology, astronomy, mathematics). Complexity, or *complexus* meaning 'braided together', can therefore be defined as a science as opposed to a theory; a science that provides a conceptual framework, a way of seeing the world which can help us make sense of things. The aim here is to review the evolving nature of healthcare education, with its focus on innovative styles of learning, and the need for a rigorous framework to address new educational challenges. Before looking at this, however, there is a need to explain what is meant by Complexity. The approach taken here is therefore two-fold: to develop a deeper understanding of Complexity and to look at how Complexity relates to healthcare education using a case study.

KEY POINTS

- Healthcare education is the process of developing a professional group using appropriate 'systems' conducive to the health of individuals, groups, and society.
- Complexity theory is an amalgam of theories arising from a range of natural sciences studying complex, dynamic phenomena.
- Complexity theory is relevant to healthcare education because it challenges educators to enable not just competence but also capability, i.e. a focus on developing the ability to creatively adapt to change and continuing professional development. Complexity therefore ensures that the delivery of healthcare keeps apace with its ever-changing context.

DISCUSSION

There are many interpretations of Complexity. A glossary would include terms such as attractor, autopoiesis, bifurcation, chaos, entropy, fractals, phase space, self organisation and so on but key to them all is the concept of 'evolving multi-dimensional systems'. These systems are therefore referred to as 'dynamic', that is, in a constant state of change with emphasis on their inter-relationships and interdependence so that they can create new order and coherence (Mittleton-Kelly, 2003). As a result of this, Complexity, unlike other theories, embeds the idea that not all phenomena can be reduced to orderly and predictable arrangements; that, in fact, physical, biological and social worlds contain phenomena that are orderly, complex and disorderly, and all exist at any one time and interact with each other. Within this perspective, complex systems exist comprising numerous interacting units that generally rely on simple rules, yet can evolve in multiple directions (Lewin, 1999; Mainzer, 2004; Waldrop,1994). It is therefore the notion of unpredictability which sets complex systems apart from simple and complicated systems (Mittleton-Kelly, 2003). This perspective makes us aware of the interactions both within and between systems and the implications this has for designing, running and evaluating educational interventions. It highlights the fact that individuals learning within systems such as the NHS change because they learn as part of an evolving process. From this perspective, the aim of any form of education is to develop not only competence, that is, relevant knowledge, skills and attitudes, but also capability to help learners deal with uncertainty and new problems as they arise, and to be able to creatively adapt to change (Cooper et al., 2004). This perspective sees learning about health and social care as an open system within a series of other inter-related systems (for example, formal learning at university or in the clinical setting, informal learning from, for example, significant others or through the Internet or media; and situational learning through personal experience) that feed back on themselves with individual reflection an on-going part of the process (Cooper and Geyer, 2008). From this perspective, the role of educators is to help learners make connections between all these different forms of learning. This perspective fits neatly within the Complexity framework.

Whilst there are many principles relating to Complexity, a number have been adapted as tools for adult education (Cooper et al., 2004; Price, 2005; Tosey, 2002). Table 6.1 shows how some of these principles have application to healthcare education. These implied Complexity principles demand that educators learn the skills of mentorship, critical reflection and self awareness and recognise that healthcare education, by its very nature, demands on-going adaptation and change for all, consumers and providers alike. This means that there is no endpoint to teaching and learning because we all evolve over time. In preparing healthcare practitioners, the end-point is not the 'perfect' nurse, doctor or physiotherapist, for instance, but a person who can continually adjust to change and recognise the need for on-going learning to address the normal changes and challenges within their working environments. To illustrate this process, a case study of research into interprofessional education (IPE) is presented.

CASE STUDY

Calls for IPE have resulted from the complex interplay of multiple interdependent systems within health and social care within which traditional 'reduce and resolve' approaches no longer work (Plesk and Grenhalgh, 2001). Such a multiple systems approach to training does not, however, fit easily into existing traditional disciplinary frameworks. This case study provides an example of how Complexity was used to guide development and evaluation of a study of IPE, funded by the Cheshire and Merseyside Strategic Health Authority in the United Kingdom. Government calls for IPE were based on the premise that it would address issues of developing

Table 6.1 Application of the principles of complexity to healthcare education (HCE)

Principle	Application	Examples
Self-organisation	Appreciation of HCE as a learning system composed of linked parts	• Create 'space' for interactive learning • Utilise electronic tools to increase availability/accessibility to target audience • Encourage cross-curricular connections
Paradox	To prepare learners for 'real life' use methods for design/delivery/evaluation that have relevance to this aim	• Promote 'connectivity' within the learning curriculum and among all the stakeholders, including users and carers • Use different educational environments to promote learning, e.g. classroom, e-learning domain, practice settings
Simple rules	Avoid over-specification of learning outcomes	• Keep learning objectives simple and general to minimise confusion • Harvest unplanned learning, e.g. learning from mistakes • Use 'problems' to guide what is needed to be known
Emergence	HCE is evolving and therefore in a constant state of change	• Be sensitive to heterogeneity in learners' levels of education, experiences, cultural values, qualifications etc. • Be aware of the effects of 'self' and of 'others' and use these as a means of role modelling
Non-linear and transformative learning	Recognise the 'teachable' moment	• Recognise that small inputs may have large effects and vice versa • Encourage 'significant event' reflections • Use previous transformative learning experiences as 'levers' for change in behaviour
Feedback	Recognise the interaction of elements within the learning system	• Recognise the inter-relationships of formal (taught), situated (practicum) and informal (social) learning • Use metaphors to explain phenomena at different levels, e.g. to aid discussion • Use peer learning to promote understanding
Connectivity	As an evolving system, focus on innovative evaluation tools to monitor processes and outcomes	• Recognise that interaction between effects may lead to unpredictable patterns that can lead eventually to transformative learning • Use quantitative and qualitative methods to evaluate outcomes and processes • Recognise that findings may differ to those expected, that incompatibilities between data sets can illuminate results, and suggest areas for change

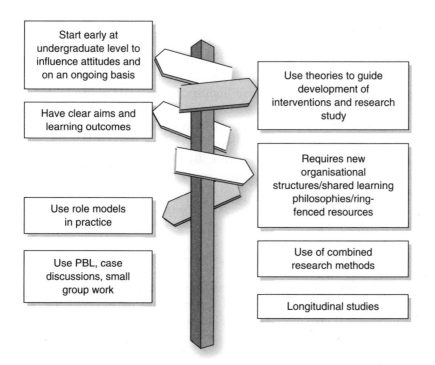

Figure 6.1 Systematic review of IPE at the undergraduate level combined with focus group research – the micro-picture of IPE

transferable skills, common discourse, cost containment, and a vehicle for political and social reform. This essentially built the macro-picture, but whilst such advice was plentiful, practical points about how to achieve it were few. As a result, a systematic review of the evidence underpinning IPE at the undergraduate level was undertaken (Cooper et al., 2001) alongside a qualitative study comprising three focus group interviews (Carlisle and Cooper, 2004). Combined findings, illustrated in Figure 6.1, highlighted the relevance of Complexity to IPE showing that it needed an interacting systems approach. This essentially built the micro-picture from which to work and led us down a pathway of integrating a multi-disciplinary lecture with self-directed e-learning in five common topics to provide a networked curriculum, interdisciplinary workshops and portfolios. The workshops were initially facilitated by a team of trained practitioners and later co-facilitated with 16 trained service users. The aim, kept simple in line with Complexity, was to develop teamwork capability.

Findings

Outcomes were evaluated using validated questionnaires, and the learning process was examined using students' narratives, focus groups and semi-structured interviews. Significant findings (analysis of covariance) showed that it enabled students to learn from each other (p<0.0001), it raised awareness about collaborative practice (p=0.03) and its link to improving care delivery (p=0.005), but not the acquisition of teamworking skills (p=0.2). Qualitative data supported these findings, highlighting students' failures to link theory to practice. To overcome this, the second cycle introduced specially trained service users into the workshops. Findings showed that through exposure to their perspectives, first-year students began to learn and apply the principles of teamwork. By placing the service user at the centre of the care process, they made connections between theory and 'real life' experiences. Findings also revealed benefits for facilitators and service users (Cooper and Spencer-Dawes, 2006; Cooper et al., 2005; Varga-Atkins and Cooper, 2005).

Lessons learnt

Complexity underpinned the study and provided the framework for drawing all the evidence together. It supplied a common discourse, giving the study interprofessional credibility by providing a 'language' for analysis and dissemination. It supported innovative and creative teaching practices with a focus on blended learning, and inclusive evaluation methods. It showed that teachers were essentially 'mentors' on the learning journey and the main 'actor' was the service user, their 'stories' brought the theory to life, illustrating how things connect. The study proved that small inputs can have large effects (butterfly effect) by providing a memorable learning experience. Finally, it provided the vehicle for validating educational reform within the institution.

CONCLUSION

What this case study showed is that Complexity provides a framework that has implicit sensitivity for education's complex nature and a satisfactory language to describe such learning in philosophical, theoretical and research terms. It provides a rigorous framework to address new educational challenges that flourish within healthcare education today.

See also: clinical competence; curriculum planning and development; interprofessional learning; partnership working; service user and carer involvement

FURTHER READING

Cooper, H. and Geyer, R. (2007) *Riding the Diabetes Roller Coaster: A New Perspective for Patients, Carers and Health Professionals.* Oxford: Radcliffe Publishing.
Sweeney, K. and Griffiths, F. (eds) (2002) *Complexity and Healthcare: An Introduction.* Oxford: Radcliffe Publishing.

key concepts in healthcare education

REFERENCES

Brew, A. (2001) *The Nature of Research: Inquiry in Academic Contexts.* London: Routledge Falmer Press.

Carlisle, C. and Cooper, H. (2004) '"Do none of you talk to each other?" The challenges facing the implementation of interprofessional education', *Medical Teacher*, 26 (6): 545–52.

Cooper, H. and Geyer, R. (2008) 'Using "complexity" for improving educational research in health care', *Social Science and Medicine*, 67: 177–82.

Cooper, H. and Spencer-Dawes, E. (2006) 'Involving service users in interprofessional education narrowing the gap between theory and practice', *Journal of Interprofessional Care*, 20 (6): 603–17.

Cooper, H., Braye, S. and Geyer, R. (2004) 'Complexity and interprofessional education', *Learning in Health and Social Care*, 3 (4): 179–89.

Cooper, H., Carlisle, C., Watkins, C. and Gibbs, T. (2001) 'Developing an evidence base for interdisciplinary learning', *Journal of Advanced Nursing*, 35 (2): 228–37.

Cooper, H., Spencer-Dawes, E. and McLean, E. (2005) 'Beginning the process of teamwork: design, implementation and evaluation of an inter-professional education intervention', *Journal of Interprofessional Care*, 19 (5): 492–508.

Lewin, R. (1999) *Complexity: Life at the Edge of Chaos*, 2nd edn. Chicago: University of Chicago Press.

Mainzer, K. (2004) *Thinking in Complexity: The Computational Dynamics of Matter, Mind, and Mankind*, 4th edn. Berlin: Springer.

Mittleton-Kelly, E. (ed.) (2003) *Complex Systems and Evolutionary Perspectives on Organisations: The Application of Complexity Theory to Organisations.* Oxford: Pergamon.

Plsek, P. and Greenhalgh, T. (2001) 'Complexity science: the challenge of complexity in health care', *British Medical Journal*, 323: 625–8.

Plsek, P.E. and Wilson, T. (2001) 'Complexity science: complexity, leadership, and management in healthcare organisations', *British Medical Journal*, 323: 746–9.

Price, J. (2005) 'Complexity and interprofessional education', in H. Colyer, M. Helme and I. Jones (eds), *The Theory–Practice Relationship in Interprofessional Education.* Higher Education Academy Health Sciences and Practice Occasional Paper No. 7, pp. 76–85.

Ross, A. (2000) *Curriculum: Construction and Critique.* London: Routledge Falmer Press.

Tosey, P. (2002) *Teaching on the Edge of Chaos: Complexity Theory and Teaching Systems.* LTSN Imaginative Curriculum Knowledge Development paper. Retrieved from LTSN website: www.ltsn.ac.uk/enhancement

Varga-Atkins, T. and Cooper, H. (2005) 'Developing e-learning for interprofessional education: testing the waters', *Telemedicine*, 11 (1): 102–4.

Waldrop, M. (1994) *Complexity: The Emerging Science at the Edge of Chaos.* Harmondsworth: Penguin.

complexity theory

33

7 curriculum models and design

Janice Gidman

key concepts in healthcare education

DEFINITION

The term 'curriculum' originated from the Latin word for 'racecourse', but evolved to mean a course incorporating the content, order and process of learning (Learning and Teaching Support Network (LTSN), 2002). Within Higher Education (HE), the term is often used with several different meanings and there are a range of definitions (Uys and Gwerle, 2005). Kelly (2004) outlines a range of aspects pertaining to the curriculum, which are summarised in Table 7.1. These aspects of the curriculum are of particular pertinence to healthcare education. The following questions should be considered by educators, in both university and practice settings:

- What differences are there (if any) between the planned and received curricula?
- What is the nature of the hidden curriculum?
- What is the nature of the informal curriculum?

KEY POINTS

- The concept of curriculum is not clearly defined and incorporates a range of aspects.
- Curriculum development is underpinned by educational philosophy.
- Professional programmes in healthcare are complex and therefore require curricula that are continually evolving.
- Content- and process-based models of curriculum development need to be integrated in the development of professional programmes.
- Constructive alignment is an essential aspect of curriculum development.

DISCUSSION

Curriculum design

Curriculum design is a major undertaking and should be viewed as a continuous developmental process, not as a one-off event (Uys and Gwerle, 2005).

Table 7.1 Aspects of the curriculum

Aspect	Description
Total curriculum	Philosophy, purpose, outcomes, content, teaching and learning strategies and assessment
Hidden curriculum	Implicit values underpinning the curriculum which influence student learning
Planned curriculum	Documented curriculum presented for validation
Received curriculum	Curriculum which is actually delivered to students – may be consciously or subconsciously modified by lecturers
Formal curriculum	Formal, timetabled learning opportunities
Informal curriculum	Informal, unplanned learning opportunities

Source: Adapted from Kelly, 2004

This needs to be considered in the context of healthcare, which is ever-changing, involves a range of professionals and service users and is increasingly complex in nature. Curriculum design should be 'a deliberate and systematic process in which learning intentions are explicit and the activities, content and assessment that promote learning are clearly aligned to and support these intentions' (LTSN, 2002: 3). The LTSN (2002) has stated that good curriculum design is central to promoting student learning and that it should:

- be underpinned by an explicit philosophy or rationale.
- be a holistic process with all aspects clearly linked and with clear progression.
- engage students in active learning to promote deep and critical approaches.
- be informed by pedagogical research.

Curriculum design must also demonstrate full consideration of academic standards and ensure that appropriate learning opportunities are available for students (Quality Assurance Agency (QAA), 2006). In the United Kingdom (UK), the QAA (2006) has published a framework to describe the achievement of awards at different taxonomical levels to ensure that programme outcomes are commensurate with the academic level being studied.

Philosophies of education and learning theories

It is evident that effective curriculum design requires consideration of the philosophies and theories that underpin the process of education. HE programmes often adopt student-centred approaches to learning and assessment. These have been influenced by the seminal works of Freire (1970) and Illich (1971), who proposed humanistic approaches to learning and argued that empowerment should be a purpose of the education process. However, it has to be acknowledged that education programmes for healthcare need to produce competent practitioners to ensure patient safety and public protection. There has been a longstanding debate within professional education as to the relative emphasis on competence and skills acquisition and on personal development and empowerment. The competency approach has led to concern that professional programmes may become reductionist in nature and lose their holistic focus (Scott, 2008; Talbot, 2004). However, government and professional publications also recognise the need to prepare autonomous professionals who can act independently in decision making (Mailloux, 2006). It is apparent that curriculum design in healthcare is a complex process that needs to incorporate both competence and personal development.

Learning theories of particular relevance to professional programme development include behavioural, cognitive, experiential, humanist, reflective and transformative learning theories. In addition to these contemporary theories, the recently emerging Complexity theory is gaining credibility as a complementary framework to support professional education (Gidman, 2009).

CONSTRUCTIVE ALIGNMENT

Biggs (2005) is attributed with developing the concept of constructive alignment, which has been widely adopted within HE. He presents a constructivist approach to education, which is consistent with student-centred learning. Constructive alignment addresses the integration of the curriculum in respect of teaching methods, assessment strategies, relationships with students, and the learning environment. Biggs (2005) contends that constructive alignment 'starts with the notion that the learner constructs his or her own learning through relevant learning activities. The teacher's job is to create a learning environment that supports the learning activities appropriate to achieving the desired learning outcomes' (2005: 1). It is essential, therefore, to ensure that all aspects of learning and teaching are aligned to each other. Biggs states that this involves:

1   identification of clear learning outcomes.
2   appropriate assessment tasks to directly assess each of the learning outcomes.
3   appropriate learning opportunities for students to be successful in assessment tasks.

Widening participation is an important aspect of HE in the UK (Department for Education and Skills, 2003) and it is essential to ensure that curriculum design is inclusive to meet the needs of the diverse student population accessing healthcare programmes. Recent years have also seen the globalisation of HE in relation to political, economic and societal trends and, in this context, universities have increasingly sought overseas markets to expand their business. It is evident that the globalisation and internationalisation of HE adds further complexity to effective curriculum design. Altbach and Knight (2007) caution that curricula designed for overseas programmes must benefit the public as well as providing an additional source of income for universities.

Table 7.2 Application of content- and process-curriculum models to concepts of healthcare education

Concept	Content-based curriculum models	Process-based curriculum models
Primary purpose of the curriculum	Focus on the acquisition of professional knowledge	Focus on personal and professional development
Definition of competence	Narrow view of competence – technical expertise – instrumental competence	Broad view of competence – holistic – relational competence
Nature of professional knowledge	Focus on academic disciplines, e.g. physiology, sociology, psychology	Focus on the integration of knowledge and application to practice
	Focus on clinical/technical skills performance	Focus on application of knowledge to skills development
Role of the student	Passive receiver of knowledge	Active learner – fully engaged with learning process
Role of the lecturer	'Expert' – passing on knowledge to students	Facilitator of learning
	Lecturer has the power in the relationship	Student and lecturer are equal partners in the relationship
Prominent theories	Behavioural and cognitive learning theories	Experiential, reflective, constructivist and transformational learning theories
Prominent teaching/ learning strategies	Didactic methods, e.g. lectures, demonstrations	Student-centred approaches, e.g. problem-based learning, reflection

Source: Adapted from Scott, 2008; Uys and Gwerle, 2005

Curriculum models

Curriculum models are generally considered to adopt either a content-based or process-based approach to curriculum development. Within content-based approaches, the HEI institution selects and controls the content of the curriculum, which is effective in terms of the time needed to deliver the programme. However, this provides limited student engagement with the learning process, which may lead to superficial learning. Process-based approaches, in contrast, are student-centred; they promote active learning by the students, which leads to deeper learning and personal development. However, this approach is time-consuming, may cover less material and lecturers need to be well prepared to facilitate learning. Table 7.2 illustrates the application of these two approaches to healthcare education.

Uys and Gwerle (2005) also refer to outcome-based approaches, which are becoming increasingly popular in professional education. They suggest that outcome-based approaches may bridge the gap between vocational and academic education and ensure skills development. However, they advise that this approach needs careful planning to prevent a narrow focus or fragmentation of learning. There is a wide range of curriculum models available for healthcare educators (see Further Reading).

CASE STUDY

This case study reflects on the author's experience of designing and delivering a curriculum for continuing professional development (CPD) in a hospital in Uganda. A team of healthcare professionals and educators, working closely with the senior nurse and principal tutor from the hospital, had previously identified the development needs of the senior nursing staff. It was evident that many of the issues identified reflected those of CPD programmes in the UK, for example the need for education on mentorship and leadership. It was essential to ensure that the programme achieved the agreed learning outcomes, whilst also meeting the specific needs of the context and culture in which it was to be delivered. This required careful consideration and on-going adaptation of the content, teaching approaches and assessment strategies, in response to the student group. This was an invaluable experience for the author and confirmed the added complexity of curriculum design and delivery within an international context – one size definitely does not fit all!

CONCLUSION

It is evident that curriculum design in healthcare programmes is a complex process that needs to be done effectively in order to promote student learning. The development of professional programmes needs to respond to the rapidly changing contexts of health and social care. Curriculum design, therefore, requires a combination of outcome- and process-based models to ensure the development of profession-specific knowledge and competence and to promote personal development and lifelong learning.

See also: assessment; behavioural learning theories; cognitive learning theories; complexity theory; curriculum planning and development; diversity and equality; humanist learning theories; quality assurance and enhancement; reflection; transformative learning

FURTHER READING

Keating, S.B. (2006) *Curriculum Development and Evaluation in Nursing.* Philadelphia: Lippincott.

Quality Assurance Agency (2008) *The Qualifications Framework for England, Wales and Northern Ireland.* Retrieved from QAA website: www.qaa.ac.uk/academicinfrastructure/FHEQ/EWNI08/default.asp

REFERENCES

Altbach, P.G. and Knight, J. (2007) 'The internationalization of higher education: motivations and realities', *Journal of Studies in International Education*, 11: 290. doi: 10.1177/1028315307303542

Biggs, J. (2005) *Aligning Teaching for Constructing Learning*. Retrieved from the HEA website: www.heacademy.ac.uk/assets/York/documents/resources/resourcedatabase/id477_aligning_teaching_for_constructing_learning.pdf

Department for Education and Skills (2003) *Widening Participation in Higher Education*. London: Department for Education and Skills.

Freire, P. (1970) *Pedagogy of the Oppressed*. London: Penguin.

Gidman, J. (2009) A Phenomenological Investigation of Pre-qualifying Nursing, Midwifery and Social Work Students' Perceptions of Learning in Practice. Unpublished PhD thesis, University of Liverpool.

Illich, I. (1971) *Deschooling Society*. New York: Marion Boyers.

Kelly, A.V. (2004) *The Curriculum Theory and Practice*, 5th edn. London: Sage.

Learning and Teaching Support Network (LTSN) (2002) *The Imaginative Curriculum*. Retrieved from the HEA website: www.heacademy.ac.uk/resources/detail/id46_The_Imaginative_Curriculum

Mailloux, C.G. (2006) 'The extent to which students' perceptions of faculties' teaching strategies, students' context and perceptions of learner empowerment predict perceptions of autonomy in BSN students', *Nurse Education Today*, 26 (7): 578–85.

Quality Assurance Agency (2006) *Code of Practice for the Assurance of Academic Quality and Standards in Higher Education. Section 7: Programme Design, Approval, Monitoring and Review*, 2nd edn. Retrieved from the QAA website: www.qaa.ac.uk/academicinfrastructure/codeofpractice/section7/

Scott, S.D. (2008) 'New professionalism – shifting relationships between nursing education and nursing practice', *Nurse Education Today*, 28 (2): 240–5.

Talbot, M. (2004) 'Monkey see, monkey do: a critique of the competency model in graduate medical education', *Medical Education*, 38 (6): 587–92.

Uys, L.R. and Gwerle, N.S. (2005) *Curriculum Development in Nursing. Process and Innovation*. London: Routledge.

8 curriculum planning and development

Ann Bryan

DEFINITION

Curriculum planning and development is one of the most creative and dynamic activities undertaken by healthcare educationalists. The production of a curriculum is a major undertaking and cannot be seen as an individual task, but rather as an on-going process. However, unless there is an initial, well-planned document that can be communicated to all those involved with the learning experience, future programme needs cannot be adapted in response to continuous evaluation of the curriculum and healthcare developments.

Traditionally, a curriculum was defined as an articulation of a framework of beliefs and knowledge that enables us to explain educational ideas. Currently, there is a much wider perspective and it is now seen to embrace all planned learning experiences. Keating, for example, defines a curriculum as 'a formal plan of study that provides the philosophical underpinnings, goals and guidelines for the delivery of a specific educational programme' (2006: 2).

The purpose of healthcare curriculum planning and development is to meet the demands of the healthcare system, the agencies responsible for educational and professional standards, lecturing staff and prospective students. All these stakeholders have their own programme requirements and if these expectations are not satisfied, the success of the curriculum could be undermined. Educationalists planning healthcare curricula have an obligation to act in the best interests of the stakeholders. Hence, the importance of effective curriculum planning and development cannot be overestimated.

KEY POINTS

- Effective stakeholder involvement is essential to successful curriculum design.
- All elements in curriculum planning and development process are linked.
- Curriculum design is subject to both internal and external pressures.
- Curriculum planning and development is a dynamic process.

DISCUSSION

In this discussion, the major issues influencing curriculum planning and development will be reviewed. The potential importance of internal and external factors that impact on it will also be highlighted and the effect they have on the delivery of successful healthcare education. Finally, it will be demonstrated that all the elements in the curriculum planning and development process are interrelated and not separate stages.

Stakeholder involvement in curriculum planning and development

Curriculum development was originally a process in which educationalists produced a validated document before consulting with stakeholders. However, contemporary approaches necessitate collaborative working with appropriate stakeholders to produce a new curriculum. Collaboration can be very beneficial, bringing creativity and innovation to the planning and development process (Lawson, 2004). The formation of a programme curriculum planning team should therefore include potential employer and student representation as well as subject and educational experts, learning resource support and service user and carer involvement, thus ensuring the optimum combination of skills and expertise.

The Leitch (2006) review has set the challenge to Higher Education Institutions (HEIs) in England of increasing the number of adults reaching graduate status to 40%. Owing to the demographic decrease of 18-year-olds in the population, this has necessitated the implementation of a widening participation strategy throughout the HEI sector. The introduction of Foundation Degrees, which include a compulsory element of work-based learning (Quality Assurance Agency (QAA), 2004), has been the main vehicle for facilitating this strategy. As Drake and Blake (2009) state, this has introduced employers who would not ordinarily engage with HEIs to the concept of university study. These partnerships between employers and universities involve working together on curriculum design, validation and review.

A number of challenges facing employers and universities have been highlighted by Reeve and Gallacher (2005). These include a lack of employer engagement, cultural differences in the partnership and quality control issues. Healthcare education has not been immune to the challenges. For example, in the late 1990s in the United Kingdom, some nursing curricula were criticised as being not 'fit for purpose' and therefore failing to produce nurses who were 'fit for practice'(Department of Health, 1997). However, this situation has improved over the past decade with increased employer input into curriculum planning and development, improvement in the relevance and quality of work-based learning, and the introduction of educational and professional benchmarking standards and practice competencies into curriculum documentation.

Strong leadership is an essential component of successful collaboration as the process can sometimes be protracted and difficult. All team members must be given the opportunity to put forward their thoughts and concerns in a non-threatening environment so as to facilitate the development of strategies that will encourage the exchange of ideas and decision making. Johnson (2006) notes that the six Cs of Lancaster's formula for collaborative research can be applied to the process of curriculum planning: through commitment, compatibility, communication and contribution, leading to consensus and credit for accomplishment, a strong leader can ensure the promotion of a successful curriculum.

Keogh et al. (2009), in their qualitative research study reviewing stakeholder involvement in the curriculum process, found some participants felt that being part of the planning team was time-consuming and had an adverse effect on their everyday work. Therefore, it is essential that the leader ensures the commitment of time, energy and resources to the undertaking. This will not only enable the contributors to prioritise curriculum planning and development but will also reinforce the value of the endeavour.

The process of curriculum planning and development

Once the appropriate contributors to the curriculum planning team have been identified, it is then necessary to formulate a robust curriculum plan. There are a number of key elements to be addressed including: context, philosophy, organisational framework and the overall aims and objectives of the programme, which together form the macro curriculum and serve as a master plan for placing content into the curriculum. It is also necessary to develop the micro curriculum, which includes module content, teaching and learning strategies, assessment and evaluation processes. The process of organising all these elements into a logical sequence is known as curriculum design. Although all steps in the sequence need to be completed, they do not need to be realised in any specific order provided that each component is thoroughly analysed so as to ensure the integrity and quality of the programme.

In the past decade external pressures have had a steadily growing influence on the curriculum planning and development process. These pressures, to a certain extent, are dictating the decisions that curriculum designers traditionally made for themselves (Learning and Teaching Support Network, 2009). Academic curriculum teams are having to assimilate the needs of various external bodies while upholding their own underpinning beliefs, values and attitudes concerning healthcare education and professional processes. The impact of this tension between internal and external influences will inevitably have implications for the planning and development cycle of the programme. In particular, it will affect the philosophy and rationale that underpin the context and foundations of the curriculum.

In the first instance, the philosophy, rationale and educational model (see the previous concept, 'Curriculum planning and development') of a prospective programme will need to be agreed at faculty level and fit, whenever possible, with the validating HEI's corporate mission statement and philosophy. This is a complicated undertaking as each curriculum planning team member will hold their own personal philosophical beliefs on what is valued in the curriculum, for example, teaching and learning theories, diversity issues and healthcare practice. It is vital that a philosophical statement is agreed by all contributing stakeholders so that what is currently valued will serve as a platform for all other curriculum components and outcomes.

One concrete result from the process of programme design is the production of a programme specification. This is used to inform the design of a programme and detail the aims and intended outcomes. Since the publication of the Dearing Report (National Committee of Inquiry into Higher Education (NCIHE), 1997), there have been a number of developments affecting the context of HE. Programme specifications are now being used for a wider range of purposes as well as providing more detailed information to students, staff, external examiners, employers and other interested parties. In particular, the QAA audit process in the UK has placed responsibility for the maintenance of standards and assurance of quality on the HEIs themselves (QAA, 2006), who are increasingly using programme specifications to provide the essential core documentation in the curriculum planning and development process.

Mapping and Benchmarking

One of the important objectives of the QAA has been to encourage the use of subject benchmark statements when designing a new programme. This external pressure has had a steadily growing influence on the curriculum planning and development process and to a certain extent prescribes many elements of a programme.

According to QAA guidelines (2006), the main purpose of subject benchmarking is to promote deep thinking on the learning that a curriculum is intended to encourage rather than set up a content-based curriculum or a draft programme specification. However, Houghton (2002) maintains that benchmark statements can be very prescriptive, particularly in relation to assessment coverage. He further argues that this is neither reasonable nor realistic. Yet, in current healthcare curriculum design subject benchmark statements are used effectively as an aid to reflection and as a mapping device against which the programme specification is justified during the validation process.

Validation and on-going currency

Traditionally, individual universities were responsible for their own quality assurance procedures. However, with the development of the QAA a more robust mechanism has been introduced which offers guidelines to support self regulation of the quality assurance process. The programme validation event within the HE sector still involves peer appraisal to ensure the quality assurance of a programmes, but now requires external reviewers to oversee the process of scrutinising all curriculum documentation.

Healthcare programmes, with the professional and practice elements that confer eligibility for registration, involve representatives from the professional organisations at validation events as well as academic staff. This creates a very different culture and ethos to the one HE validation committees originally intended. The marked diversity of membership of the validation committee amplifies the capacity for differences regarding values, views and experiences. These variances can be viewed positively since the need for representation from all interested parties ensures the legitimacy of the decisions made by the validation committee.

Once the validation committee decision has been endorsed by the HEI governing body and the programme has been validated, it is necessary to review the curriculum on a regular basis so that it maintains currency. Within healthcare education, evaluation of the curriculum and programme is through the systematic collection of data, which can result in minor or major modifications by the appropriate quality assurance committee. It is essential when making improvements to ensure that all elements of the curriculum maintain their cohesion. No one element should be changed without considering the impact on the overall curriculum design.

CASE HISTORY

The University was commissioned to write a Postgraduate Certificate in Clinical Case Management for a new community matron role. A curriculum planning committee was formed by the Faculty curriculum lead, including academics, library and support services, employer and student representatives and a user organisation member. Over a two-month period the philosophy, rationale, programme specification, module descriptors and management document were vigorously debated and prepared for a validation event. The programme was successfully validated. However, it needed adjustments within six months of the validation event owing to the introduction of new government case management benchmarks and the on-going evaluation of the curriculum as the community matron's role evolved. Hence, a major modification of the curriculum was undertaken and the programme mapped to new subject benchmarks. This ensured that the curriculum not only maintained its currency, but also determined further commissions from the appropriate authorities.

CONCLUSION

Curriculum planning and development are a major responsibility for healthcare educationalists. Various internal and external factors need to be taken into account within the context of the HEI's quality structure as well as the philosophical beliefs of the faculty. Careful planning and strong leadership are necessary to ensure effective communication between stakeholders so that the curriculum meets the needs of all interested parties. The curriculum document itself should never be regarded as a finished product, but should always form the basis for further revision and development.

See also: curriculum models and design; leadership and management in academia; partnership working; quality assurance and enhancement

FURTHER READING

Keating, S. (2006) *Curriculum Development and Evaluation in Nursing*. Philadelphia: Lippincott, Williams and Wilkins.

REFERENCES

Department of Health (1997) *Project 2000: Fitness for Purpose Report*. London: Department of Health.

Drake, J. and Blake, J. (2009) 'Employer engagement: the critical role of employee commitment', *Education and Training*, 1 (1): 23–42.

Houghton, W. (2002) 'Using QAA subject benchmark information: an academic teacher's perspective', *Quality Assurance in Education*, 10 (3): 172–86.

Johnson, J. (2006) 'Responsibilities of Faculty in Curriculum Development and Evaluation', in S. Keating (ed.), *Curriculum Development and Evaluation in Nursing*. Philadelphia: Lippincott, Williams and Wilkins. pp. 31–45.

Keating, S. (2006) *Curriculum Development and Evaluation in Nursing*. Philadelphia: Lippincott, Williams and Wilkins.

Keogh, J., Fourie, W., Watson, J. and Gay, H. (2009) 'Involving the stakeholders in the curriculum process: a recipe for success?', *Nurse Education Today*, 30 (1): 37–43.

Lawson, H. (2004) 'The logic of collaboration in education and the human services', *Journal of Inter-professional Care*, 18 (3): 225–37.

Learning and Teaching Support Network (2009) Retrieved from HEA website: www.heacademy.ac.uk/assets/York/documents/resources/resourcedatabase/id57_contexts_for_curriculum_design_working_with_external_pressures.rtf

Leitch, S. (2006) *Prosperity for All in the Global Economy – World Class Skills*. Norwich: HMSO.

NCIHE (1997) *National Committee of Inquiry into Higher Education* (Dearing Report). Norwich: HMSO.

Quality Assurance Agency (2004) *Foundation Degree: Qualification Bench Mark*. Gloucester: Quality Assurance Agency for Higher Education.

Quality Assurance Agency (2006) *Guidelines for Programme Specifications*. Retrieved from QAA website: www.qaa.ac.uk/academicinfrastructure/programSpec/guidelines06.pdf

Reeve, F. and Gallacher, J. (2005) 'Employer–university partnerships: a key problem for work-based learning programmes?', *Journal of Education and Work*, 18 (2): 219–33.

9 dealing with failing and problem students

Julie Williams

DEFINITION

The definition of the term 'fail', according to the Oxford English Dictionary (2009), is being unsuccessful in an undertaking, being unable to meet standards, neglecting to do something or disappointing expectations. In the context of healthcare education, a student could be failing to achieve either academically, clinically (including competence and professional attributes) or on a personal level.

A 'problem' is defined as an unwelcome or harmful matter needing to be dealt with (Oxford English Dictionary, 2009). In healthcare programmes this can include students who exhibit disruptive behaviour, fail to engage with the educational process, lack motivation or influence others negatively; it also includes factors relating to professional elements including being unsafe in practice or professional unsuitability.

KEY POINTS

- There is a major focus on the progression and retention of students, especially in relation to pre-qualifying healthcare programmes.
- Robust recruitment and admission procedures are essential to support candidates and to ensure that students' expectations are realistic.
- The motivation of students can play a key role in determining their failure or success.
- Regular progress reviews enable early identification of underachievement and provide the opportunity for additional support.
- Effective preparation for practice is important to reduce students' anxiety.

DISCUSSION

Failing students

In recent years, much attention has been paid to the progression and attrition rates of students in healthcare, especially in relation to undergraduate pre-registration programmes of study. Reasons for failure are various and often interlinked: as Glogowska et al. (2007) noted, attrition amongst students in healthcare is usually down to more than one factor. Failing to achieve success and make suitable progress can be as a result of failing to reach the required minimum standard of either, or both, academic and practice competencies. In addition, there may be significant personal reasons why students underachieve, such as financial difficulties, ill health, family commitments, or they may decide they have embarked on a programme of study they are not suited to. There is much that a Higher Education Institution (HEI) can do in relation to enhancing student progression and retention. As McSherry and Marland (1999) stated, HEIs should establish models of best practice and operate mechanisms for dealing with the processes involved in the failure of students.

Recruitment and admission procedures must sufficiently support applicants and the management of student expectations is an important matter. Students need to know, and be clear about, what they can expect, what the extent and limitations of the provision are and be assured that they will be treated fairly and equitably. Strategies such as pre-admission literacy and numeracy assessments and diagnostic assessment can help in the early detection and recognition of the need for increased support for some students. Pre-programme criminal record checks (with subsequent annual declarations), and occupational health assessments can help determine individual suitability and fitness to practise as a healthcare student.

Students should be formatively and summatively assessed, and have regular reviews of their progress, at strategic points throughout their studies. The provision of constructive feedback on their endeavours is of crucial importance to the students. Therefore, debriefing and feedback on progress are important elements of support for anyone involved with an underachieving student.

The motivation of students can play a key role in determining their failure or success. There is no single theoretical interpretation of motivation and there are many factors that determine whether students will be motivated to learn or not. As Hoskins and Newstead (2009) noted, the extent to which students want to succeed can result in motivated or amotivated behaviours; they recommended ascertaining motivation through specifically designed tasks and encouraging motivation through an effective learning context and the provision of good quality feedback. Some students may hide their vulnerabilities and anxieties by assuming deliberate and calculated approaches to their studies, looking as if they understand when, in fact, they do not. Such surface approaches to learning can have a negative effect and students may consequently do the bare minimum in order to get the desired grade. These students may become disengaged from their learning and, eventually, be more unlikely to seek the help they need, thus erecting more barriers to their achievement and progression. These can manifest in, for example, numerous applications for deferral of assessment submission dates or, in some cases, non-submissions.

Research by Robshaw and Smith (2003) showed that student nurses in their study stayed on the programme, despite struggling academically and coping with financial or personal difficulties, because of a desire to succeed that overrode all the transient problems. Learning and teaching relationships therefore need to acknowledge the students' perspective and provide encouragement and positive reinforcement on a holistic level, fostering motivation and progression where possible.

Within both practice and educational settings, mentors and teachers need to be aware of the significant commitment required by all participants when contributing to student learning, achievement and progression. In an ideal world, students would be engaged in a mutually positive relationship with those facilitating their learning. However, in the actual world, things may be different and some students experience dissonance with previously held expectations. For example, what is reflected in everyday practice may, and often does, reveal a very different ideal (Duffy, 2003). Thus, failing to progress in either theoretical or clinical endeavours may be as a result of students' preconceived and unmatched expectations. Regular reviews of progress with personal academic tutors can help counter any potential problems and provide opportunities for additional pastoral support.

Educational programme teams should develop strong relationships with placement partners in order to support link lecturers, mentors and students in their respective roles. Duffy (2003) suggested that lecturers should play a key role in the conduct of practice assessments of student nurses and contribute to supporting all those involved with the difficult task of failing a student who is underachieving in practice, especially in relation to attitudes.

There is an enduring concern with students being sufficiently prepared for their placements. The introduction of simulated learning and skills laboratories has significantly increased opportunities to develop and demonstrate competence in practice skills prior to starting a placement. Early recognition of students' learning needs and potential deficits enables individual action plans to be developed with a focus on the requisite minimum standards to be achieved in relation to knowledge, skills and attitudes. Mentors and students can then work together in the completion and achievement of these individualised learning plans, with a clear focus on the required outcomes, the processes and the time scales necessary for success.

Problem students

Students with disruptive behaviour patterns present problems for those managing the student group. It is not unreasonable to ask a disruptive student to leave the room. Students who persistently arrive late, or fail to arrive at all, should be counselled and helped to devise personal strategies for dealing with these problems, after determining there are no causative factors that require occupational health and medical intervention. Students who display negative attitudes towards staff and service users and who, despite advice and support, continue to fail in their understanding, or performance, of professional requirements, may find themselves subject to the judgement of a professional suitability panel which may invoke a termination of studies for the student concerned. There are various strategies that can be employed to deal with problem students.

Where a student lacks the motivation to engage in their education, reasons for their disengagement should be sought; educators should ensure that students know what they need to do, how to proceed, and how to determine when they have achieved success. Determining the ways in which any negative situations can be rectified, finding compromise and, most importantly, helping students learn from the experiences are core in the process for educators. This includes empowering students to take responsibility for their actions and concluding with positive observations, examples or praise. Such practices call for assertiveness and careful management of any differences in opinion.

Where conflict does occur, the educator should reflect on its cause, make plans to deal with it, and document all observations, outcomes, behaviours and lessons learned. Unresolved conflict can negatively influence the student's learning experience and that of others, and should not be ignored. The HEI's support facilities can be accessed to help in resolving some problems, but students who fail to make the requisite progression, for whatever reason, should be helped to find an alterative pathway for their future studies and/or career choices.

At times, there can be incidences of academic malpractice to be dealt with, one of the most common being plagiarism. Institutional policies and procedures must be clearly laid down and accessible to all students at the beginning of their studies. Clear teaching and learning strategies to enhance student academic writing and literacy are essential, as it is not unusual for students to claim to be unaware that they have plagiarised work. Harper (2006) noted that, while research in this area is sparse, the evidence does suggest that dishonesty in academic settings can translate to dishonest and unethical behaviour in practice settings, opining that addressing such issues may help prevent misconduct in the healthcare professions. On a positive note, research by Ahrin and Jones (2009) showed that, while it is the case that some students in healthcare are involved in academic malpractice, sometimes unperceived or unintentional, the students in their study were more aware of behaviours that were academically dishonest, compared to students from other disciplines.

Ultimately, as McSherry and Marland (1999) opined, it is unrealistic to expect that all students will successfully complete their programmes, as academic and professional standards have to be maintained and upheld; what is required is fairness and clear reasons for failure agreed for those involved. HEIs should ensure that appropriate careers advice and sources of support are offered, and known, to such students to help them in the future.

CASE STUDY

William, a student nurse, had excelled in practice, but during his final placement his mentor noticed he was late for duty on a regular basis and increasingly absent. William had become unwilling to engage with staff and patients and recently had demonstrated a lack of motivation. His mentor was concerned enough to discuss these issues with him at one of their regular progress reviews. By the time of his interim assessment, William had been absent from duty on several more occasions, inevitably affecting the opportunities to acquire, demonstrate and develop his clinical skills; he was deemed unable to meet the required learning outcomes and standards. William and his mentor agreed that he had not yet achieved the required minimal standard and had therefore failed an element of his practice assessment.

In order for William to achieve all his practice learning outcomes, a schedule of activities within a bespoke action plan was developed. Weekly meetings were planned in order to monitor and support William's progress, but despite regular support from his mentor, and others, he continued to make poor progress. The mentor contacted the HEI link lecturer to discuss the concerns. A meeting was held between William, his mentor and the link lecturer to discuss his lack of progression and how best to support the achievement of his placement learning outcomes. It transpired that William had been dealing with a family tragedy and had not felt able to ask for help. He was given some short-term compassionate leave and returned to placement where he was able to complete all of his assessments successfully.

CONCLUSION

Supporting underachieving, or problem, students must take note of their prevailing attitudes, beliefs and perceptions, as well as their individual circumstances. It involves paying attention to all aspects of the educational experience and environment, creating a strong sense of shared purpose, implementing robust support mechanisms, setting policies that are consistent with good practice and having realistic expectations for individual performance. Ultimately, whilst some students will inevitably fail, or be discontinued due to professional unsuitability or misconduct, providing a holistic approach to support of students and their educational experience can facilitate success.

See also: feedback and marking; learning environments; mentorship; role model; student support

FURTHER READING

Duffy, K. (2003) *Failing Students: A Qualitative Study of Factors that Influence the Decisions Regarding Assessment of Students' Competence in Practice.* London: NMC.

Hoskins, S.L. and Newstead, S.E. (2009) 'Encouraging student motivation', in F. Fry, S. Ketteridge and S. Marshall (eds), *A Handbook for Teaching and Learning in Higher Education*, 3rd edn. London: Routledge. pp. 27–40.

REFERENCES

Ahrin, A.O. and Jones, K.A. (2009) 'A multidiscipline exploration of college students' perceptions of academic dishonesty: are nursing students different from other college students?', *Nurse Education Today*, 29 (7): 710–14.

Duffy, K. (2003) *Failing Students: A Qualitative Study of Factors that Influence the Decisions Regarding Assessment of Students' Competence in Practice.* London: NMC.

Glogowska, M., Young, P. and Lockyer, L. (2007) 'Should I go or should I stay?', *Active Learning in Higher Education*, 8 (1): 63–77.

Harper, M. (2006) 'High tech cheating', *Nurse Education Today*, 26 (8): 672–9.

Hoskins, S.L. and Newstead, S.E. (2009) 'Encouraging student motivation', in F. Fry, S. Ketteridge and S. Marshall (eds), *A Handbook for Teaching and Learning in Higher Education*, 3rd edn. London: Routledge. pp 27–40.

McSherry, W. and Marland, G.R. (1999) 'Student discontinuations: is the system failing?', *Nurse Education Today*, 19 (7): 578–85.

Oxford English Dictionary (2009) Retrieved from the OED website: www.ask.oxford.com

Robshaw, M. and Smith, J. (2003) 'Keeping afloat: student nurses' experiences following assignment referral', *Nurse Education Today*, 24 (7): 511–20.

key concepts in healthcare education

10 diversity and equality

Elizabeth Mason-Whitehead

DEFINITION

'Equality' and 'diversity' are two terms often used interchangeably, but as the following definitions demonstrate, they represent two different experiences.

Equality is concerned with 'creating a fairer society where everyone can participate and have the opportunity to fulfil their potential' (Department of Health (DH), 2004). When we consider the definition of equality, we are mindful that our social identities of gender, disability, race, age, religion, social class and sexuality may influence every sphere of our lives. Such examples may include job promotion, entering higher education (HE) and living a long and fulfilling life.

Diversity is concerned with the notion of 'difference'. Within any society or community there are individuals and groups of people who are regarded as 'different' and such variations are frequently regarded as something that is 'discreditable' (Goffman,1963) and this may lead to them being stigmatised and discriminated against. However, diversity can also be an 'all-embracing term, where everyone works together, promoting the potential of each individual person' (Mason-Whitehead and Mason, 2007: 161).

KEY POINTS

- Issues of equality and diversity are apparent in every aspect of the experience of HE and educators must lead by example to promote a fairer society.
- Social identity is made up of our gender, race/ethnicity, sexuality, religion/faith, age and disability. Having an awareness and appreciation of how an individual's social identity may have an impact on his or her academic and clinical learning experience and engagement is an important aspect of an educator's role.
- Discrimination refers to the unfair treatment of at least one of the aspects of our social identity. Institutional discrimination refers to discrimination that is enmeshed into the structures and polices of organisations. Discrimination is often referred to as prejudice put into practice.
- Students of healthcare education reflect an increasingly diverse society and educators need to respond to the opportunities and challenges that this presents.

- The eight strands of equality legislation embrace the following; age, disability, gender, sexual orientation, race, religion/belief, human rights and carers. It is important for all those engaged in the provision of education of students that they are familiar with the legal framework relating to equality and discrimination in the country in which they are working.

DISCUSSION

The most translated document in the world is the Universal Declaration of Human Rights, which was born out of the events of the Second World War and brings together a world sentiment that there are rights to which all human beings are entitled. The following extract from Article 2 of the Declaration expresses a 60-year-old commitment which is as true today as when it was first published in 1948:

> Everyone is entitled to all rights and freedoms set forth in this Declaration, without distinction of any kind, such as race, colour, sex, language, religion, political or other opinion, national or social origin, property, birth or status. Furthermore, no distinction shall be made on the basis of the political jurisdictional or international status of the country or territory to which a person belongs, whether it be independent, trust, non-self-governing or under any other limitation of sovereignty. (Universal Declaration of Human Rights, 1948)

Most of us, in our roles in healthcare education, engage with some aspect of diversity and equality. It is embedded within every aspect of our working lives and this may include serving on a university's Diversity and Equality Committee, teaching health inequalities to nursing students or writing a contribution like this which seeks to inform and raise awareness.

Equality and diversity legislation

This section provides an overview of the legislation relating to equality and diversity. It is an essential reference for all of us working with students in HE. Clearly, countries other than the UK have different legal frameworks, but essentially the criteria of promoting diversity and working towards equality ought to remain the same. The eight strands of commonly held equality and diversity principles, as identified by the NHS Employers Organisation (2009) are as follows:

1. *Age*: The Employment Equality (Age) Regulations 2006 protects against discrimination on grounds of age in employment and vocational training.
2. *Disability*: The Disability Discrimination Act (DDA) 1995 outlaws discrimination of disabled people in employment, provision of goods, facilities and services. The Discrimination Amendment Act 2005 introduces the duty required of public bodies to promote equality for disabled people.

3. *Gender*: The Employment Equality (Sex Discrimination) Regulations 2005 prohibit discrimination on the grounds of pregnancy or the taking of maternity leave. The Equal Pay Act 1970 (Amended) gives an individual a right to the same pay and benefits as a person of the opposite sex in the same employment, where the man and woman are doing like work to be of equal value.

4. *Sexual orientation*: The Employment Equality (Sexual Orientation) Regulation 2003 protects against discrimination on the grounds of sexual orientation in employment, vocational training, promotion and working conditions. The Civil Partnerships Act 2004 provides legal recognition and parity of treatment for same-sex and married couples, including employment and pension rights. The Gender Recognition Act 2004 provides legal recognition in their acquired gender.

5. *Race and ethnicity*: There have been a number of Acts and regulations relating to race and ethnicity. The Race Relations Act 1976 prohibits discrimination in employment, education and provision of goods and services. The Act was amended in 2000 to make it a statutory duty to promote equal opportunity and promote good relations. This Act was further amended in 2003 and introduced new definitions of indirect discrimination and harassment.

6. *Religion or belief*: The Equality in Employment Regulations (Religion or Belief) 2003 directive protects against discrimination on the grounds of religion, vocational training, promotion and working conditions. The Racial and Religious Hatred Act 2006 aims to stop people from intentionally using threatening words or behaviour to stir up hatred.

7. *Carers*: A number of Acts have been introduced to protect carers from discrimination and promote equality, including: the Work and Families Act 2006; the Carers (Equal Opportunities) Act 2004; the Employment Act 2002 and the Employment Relations Act 1999.

8. *Human rights*: The Human Rights Act 1998 applies to all public authorities, making it unlawful to violate the European Convention on Human Rights.

The social identities of diversity

One of the greatest strengths of healthcare programmes of education is to be found in the diversity of their students. At the time of writing, the 'Freshers' are arriving at our university and as the weeks unfold the students will take heart from the fact that many of their new friends will share similar challenges to themselves. Typically they may be carers, lone parents, have dyslexia, experience financial difficulties, live with long-term medical conditions, such as asthma or diabetes, or just feel 'embarrassed' because they are mature students. Figure 10.1 is a reminder of the wide range of social identities which are present in every intake of new students.

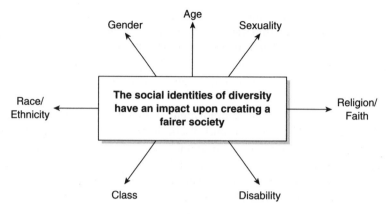

Figure 10.1   The social identities of diversity

Supporting students' diversity and their experience of learning

Supporting students is one of the most rewarding and challenging roles of educators, and the way that students are guided can determine whether or not they continue with their studies. Figure 10.2 identifies a range of ways in which students can be supported to fulfil their potential irrespective of their social identity.

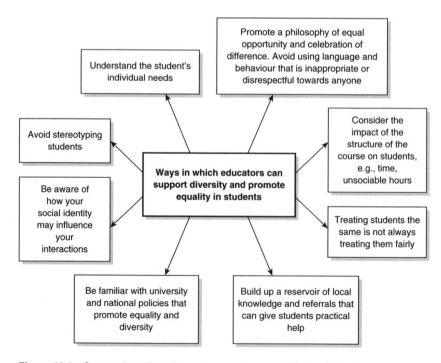

Figure 10.2   Supporting diversity and promoting equality in students

Working towards equality and promoting diversity

There have been a number of initiatives and research projects that have considered how to manage equality and cultural diversity within educational and healthcare environments. For example, Hunt (2007) offers a framework of themes that develop racial equality and cultural diversity in the health workforce. Kai (2007) considers how flexible routes into healthcare training may increase the numbers of people from ethnic minorities entering health careers. Sometimes it is identified that a particular group is under-represented. In such cases, the organisation may encourage applicants and train staff responsible for selection. This is known as *positive action* but it is not offering a job *on the basis* of gender or ethnic group, which would be illegal. Another way of promoting diversity is through *reasonable adjustment*, where an organisation makes adjustments that allow a disabled person to work. Such examples include making structural changes to the organisation's premises, providing a reader or interpreter or changing the working hours.

A report commissioned by the Equality and Human Rights Commission (2009) put forward a number of good practices for integration in the workplace found in eight UK organisations and these are summarised as follows:

- Advice booklets that gave employees and managers an insight into diverse religions or beliefs practised by colleagues and customers.
- Advice to line managers about allowing staff to take time to pray, accommodating religious festivals and balancing polices on uniform and religious requirements.
- Abolishment of the set retirement age.
- Employing diversity specialists and diversity champions at senior levels to raise awareness of equality and diversity.
- Actively implementing equality practices.
- Establishing in-house equality programmes.
- Encouraging staff networks for particular groups (such as gay and bisexual employees).
- Providing information on age discrimination.
- Adopting flexible workplace polices and implementation.
- Challenging discrimination and harassment.

Widening participation

As educators, we are committed in ensuring that the students enrolled on our programmes represent all walks of life. The Higher Education Funding Council for England (HEFCE) recognises that students leaving HE have the ability to enhance their country's development from a range of perspectives, such as their communication skills, critical thinking and ability to manage complex information. HEFCE recognises that many students are still not accessing HE and the HEFCE Strategic Plan 2006–11 sets out a range of objectives to develop widening access for potential students (HEFCE, 2009). Educators, in whatever country they work, can make a significant contribution in widening access and participation for potential students. Such initiatives include visiting schools, holding 'taster' courses, having flexible entry requirements, running part-time courses, supporting students with special educational needs and ensuring that institutes are part of the community, rather than the ivory tower at the top of the hill!

CASE STUDY

Anna is a newly appointed university lecturer who was previously employed as a nurse consultant. At her interview Anna expressed her long-standing interest in working towards equality for colleagues and patients and, if appointed, she would like to continue to develop this role. Within the first six months of her new position, Anna, with the support from the Faculty Management Team, set up a working party comprising of students, academic and practice staff and members of the public with a remit to promote equality and diversity. The newly created Equality and Diversity Group liaises closely with similar groups in the university and has a particular focus on students, employers and healthcare users. The group's specialist information on areas such as policy, education and workplace discrimination proves a valuable resource for the faculty and the university. The group, under Anna's leadership, is now launching its own quarterly journal, which serves to promote equality and diversity through education, policy and discussion.

CONCLUSION

By the time this book is published, the present trends of people living in a country other than their own, the number of students with special educational needs, the registering of disabled students and the number of students with complex health and social problems will have continued to rise steadily. Never before have the challenges and opportunities to work for equality and celebrate diversity presented themselves in HE in the way that they do now. New educators need to equip themselves with knowledge, sensitivity and creativity, and for the more 'seasoned' of us, we must accept that the world and its students are changing fast and if we are to provide the best possible learning experience for them then we have to seize the opportunity and adapt accordingly.

See also: academic staff development; dealing with failing and problem students; leadership and management in academia; learning environments; role model; specific learning needs of students

FURTHER READING

Brown-Glaude, W.B. (ed.) (2009) *Doing Diversity in Higher Education: Faculty Leaders Share Challenges and Strategies*. Brunswick, NJ: Rutgers University Press.

Cooper, D. (2004) *Challenging Diversity: Rethinking Equality and the Value of Difference*. New York: Cambridge University Press.

Graham, H. (2007) *Unequal Lives: Health and Socio-economic Inequalities*. Maidenhead: Open University Press.

REFERENCES

Department of Health (2004) *Sharing the Challenge, Sharing the Benefits – Equality and Diversity in the Medical Workforce Directorate*. London: Department of Health.

Equality and Human Rights Commission (2009) *New Workplace Report Launched*. Retrieved from the Equality and Human Rights Commission website: www.equalityhumanrights.com/media-centre/new-workplace-report

Goffman, E. (1963) *Stigma – Notes on Managing Spoiled Identity*. London: Penguin.

HEFCE (2009) *Strategic Plan 2006–11*. (Updated June 2009). Retrieved from the HEFCE website: www.hefce.ac.uk/pubs/hefce/2009/09_21

Hunt, B. (2007) 'Managing equality and cultural diversity in the health workforce', *Journal of Clinical Nursing*, 16 (12): 2252–59.

Kai, J. (2007) 'Safety and achieving equality amid diversity in health care', *British Journal of General Practice*, 57 (543): 774–6.

Mason-Whitehead, E. and Mason, T. (2007) *Study Skills for Nurses*. London: Sage.

NHS Employers Organisation (2009) *The Eight Strands of Equality*. Retrieved from the NHS Employers Organisation website: www.nhsemployers.org/EmploymentPolicyAndPractice/Equality

Universal Declaration of Human Rights (UDHR) (1948) *Article 2*. Retrieved from the Center for a World in Balance website: www.worldinbalance.net/agreements/1948-udhr.html

11 e-learning

Jill McCarthy

DEFINITION

E-learning is an all encompassing term to describe learning supported by the use of information and communication technologies. Previously referred to as computer enhanced learning, e-learning now includes the use of mobile technologies such as personal digital assistants, mobile telephones and MP3 players (Mason and Viner, 2007). It is suited to distance learning, but it can also be used in conjunction with face-to-face learning, whereby it is often referred to as blended learning. In education, it is common to create a virtual learning environment, often in conjunction with a managed information system, to develop a managed learning environment. These can support programmes through a user interface which is standard throughout an institution; an example of such an environment is Blackboard. Distance learning, flexible learning and open learning are all broader terms that incorporate e-learning, but include all instructional situations where educators and students are physically separated.

KEY POINTS

- E-learning is learning supported by information and communication technologies.
- E-learning includes the use of mobile technologies.
- When used alongside traditional teaching, it is referred to as blended learning.
- Virtual learning environments are often used to present e-learning programmes.
- E-learning is a further development of distance learning.

DISCUSSION

There is an opinion that, in the future, education will be delivered, in the main, at a distance from the learner through technology (e.g. Pausch, 2002). E-learning offers a flexible, individualised approach whereby students can proceed at their own pace, at their chosen time and within their chosen environment. However, education may be considered sluggish in taking advantage of the digital learning age, and most educational institutes still maintain central control of learning by delivering standardised courses which students attend, administering these courses with a top-down approach.

It is considered that technology could dramatically change how education is delivered by altering both the learning and teaching environment. As Siegel noted:

> No longer will the teacher disseminate information in the form of lectures and textbooks. Rather the teacher will adopt the role of facilitator, tutor, and learner. Similarly, the student's role will change from a memorizer of facts and principles to that of a researcher, problem-solver, and strategist. (2002: 2)

Using educational buildings as central contact points for learning can create problems. The educator controls the classroom, which means that they also control the time when learning takes place, the students who participate, the environment, the resources, the pace of learning, the subject matter and, in many cases, the results. Forman et al. (2002) commented that there is a prevailing, yet misguided, perception that learning takes place only when teaching is directly controlled by educators.

The impetus for the introduction of e-learning into health education is emanating from several distinct, but, interrelated factors originating from within and outside of the education sector, with educationalists having little opportunity to influence courses (McCarthy and Holt, 2007). In the United Kingdom (UK), the government is keen to increase productivity and commissioned an independent review. This established a clear link between productivity and workforce education and training, with implications for the education sector that a demand-led, as opposed to supply-led, system of education was required, with employers having a greater say in what is taught, by whom and to what level (Leitch, 2006).

Thus health educators are eager to embrace new partnerships with relevant employers, and implicit in this is the need for flexible delivery modes, in order that the workforce will not be put under further strain by staff absent from work on study leave. In the UK, the Department of Health (DH) is increasing the use of information technologies by National Health Service staff generally and this aim is to be achieved in all areas, including education (DH, 2005). Not only is the higher education sector required to teach health professionals how to use new technologies effectively, but also, it is encouraging widening participation through the more flexible approach of e-learning (E-mpirical, 2006).

The digital age is upon us and there appears to be a sudden rush to achieve online programmes within educational institutions (Lewis and Whitlock, 2003). However, there is a need to use these technologies correctly if they are to be effective; this requires skills and training and is a time-consuming endeavour. For example, it is estimated that for every hour of online learning material, there is a need for 30–200 hours of development time (Horton, 2000). Programmes have to be correctly designed to optimise student performance and both educators and learners have to be computer competent to gain maximum benefits from this style of education. Online learning brings with it a paradigm shift in terms of the role of the educator. The whole focus of learning shifts from one of teacher-centred to learner-centred (Glen and Cox, 2006) and the role of the educator changes to one of facilitator which, whilst offering benefits such as independent learning, requires the educator to be versed in this style of pedagogy. Lecturers need to be able to foster management of knowledge, and programmes need to encourage independent inquiry and not be packaged units of information. Learning via technology is a challenge to traditional styles of teaching and learning and, as Bourne et al. (1997) noted, is evolving its own science of teaching. Much of the literature on e-learning stresses the importance of interactivity in the virtual classroom and the need for group working and online communities, so that the learner is not isolated and marginalised (Moule, 2006).

Successful e-learning takes place within a complex system involving the students' experiences of learning, teachers' strategies, teachers' planning and thinking and the teaching/learning context (Glen and Cox, 2006). Students have become lifelong learners, due to fluctuations in work patterns, resulting in mixed ability and mixed age classes. Also, the surge in the use of technology for learning has brought with it a series of challenges. There are reports of educators having discovered students using mobile telephones to text answers during tests, and of students purchasing online bespoke assignments, which would ordinarily take hours of research and writing (Coll, 2007). In addition to these challenges, the intellectual property rights of online information are not always clear and debates rage, causing further confusion for educationalists.

David, aged 28, is a physiotherapist. He is married to Sally, who also works full-time, and they have one small child. David is keen to further his career and embark upon a Masters degree in Sports Science. However, although his employers have agreed to part fund his degree they cannot, because of limited staff, allow him time off from work to attend university. David has made enquiries within his region, and one university offers this programme by blended learning, consisting of a modular approach with a mixture of some weekend workshops and e-learning.

David is a little apprehensive about this style of education, feeling that he needs the dynamics of group attendance to motivate him. With this in mind he telephones the course tutor, Mary, who explains that the students usually are busy, mature professionals who are working full-time like himself. She says that she has always found the cohorts to be very motivated and encourages students to swap telephone numbers and email addresses when they first meet, in order to support one another. Mary stresses to David the importance of this peer support and of seeking help from the course team if required. She assures him that all students are well supported throughout the degree; course tutors keep in contact with students regularly, both online and by telephone. Mary explains that the e-learning part of the programme is easy to follow and will consist of clear directions, for example, instructing students to read a specific article and then reflect upon this, or to join in a discussion on the e-board about the article. Mary points out that the discussion board entries are often included as part of the module assessment and this encourages students to participate. She also explains that the e-learning is synchronous; each session is open for access for three weeks, which provides flexibility, whilst ensuring that discussions boards are current and students do not fall too far behind. She tells David that over the past three years since the programme was introduced the student attrition rate is less than with the previous traditional delivery, whilst the grades of students have been higher.

CONCLUSION

Both academia and the corporate world appear keen to embrace the new technologies of e-learning with all the advantages that this style of education can bring with it. However, as is common with new ventures, challenges are accompanying the introduction of e-learning which need to be addressed. Chozos et al. discussed the concern that, owing to lack of face-to-face contact, new policies need to be implemented in regard to 'equity, legality, privacy and justice stemming from political, social, cultural and economical implications' (2002: 1).

E-learning is in its infancy and it seems that by careful nurturing through research and development it could grow and develop successfully within health education. If e-learning is implemented with sufficient time for development, by experienced and knowledgeable educators, technicians and administrators, and if sufficient finances are allocated to its operation in order that innovative equipment can be installed to maximise capabilities, then e-learning could prove to be a success. Not only could it assist with the problem of staff shortages by aiding recruitment through flexible modes of delivery, but also it can provide flexibility in the length of time students take to qualify. E-learning offers new and exciting possibilities in health education if utilised to its full potential. Interactive environments can provide innovative and stimulating settings in which to explore health-related subjects. Online videos can broadcast lectures and presentations from anywhere in the world, by anyone, including media stars and historical figures. Imagine the interest generated in a presentation by, for example, Angelina Jolie on *International Aid*, or a discussion by Mother Theresa on *Child Malnutrition*, or, indeed, a lecture by Florence Nightingale on *The Nature of Nursing*. These scenarios are possible and, indeed, feasible through e-learning.

See also: academic staff development; assessment; diversity and equality; humanist learning theories; learning environments

FURTHER READING

Glen, S. and Moule, E. (eds) (2006) *E-learning in Nursing*. Basingstoke: Palgrave Macmillan.
Salmon, G. (2004) *Essential E-Moderating Guide for New Generation of Tutors*. Milton Keynes: Open University Press.

REFERENCES

Bourne, J.R., McMaster, E., Rieger, J. and Campbell, J.O. (1997) 'Paradigms for online learning: a case study in the design and implementation of an asynchronous learning networks (ALN) course', *Journal of Asynchronous Learning Networks*, 1 (2): 38–56.
Chozos, P., Lytras, M. and Pouloudi, N. (2002) *Ethical Issues in E-learning: Insights from the Application of Stakeholder Analysis in Three E-learning Cases*. Retrieved from www.dcs.gla.ac.uk/~nick/papers/EL_%20paper.pdf
Coll, K. (2007) 'Technological age spurs cheating', *Sidelines Online*. Retrieved from http://media.www.mtsusidelines.com/media/storage/paper202/news/2007/02/08/Features/Technological.Age.Spurs.Cheating-2707498.shtml
Department of Health (2005) *Supporting Best Practice in E-learning across the NHS*. London: Department of Health.
E-mpirical (2006) *Modernising Healthcare Training: E-learning in Healthcare Services*. Retrieved from www.nationalworkforce.nhs.uk/national%5felearning%5freport%5fmay06.pdf
Forman, D., Nyatanga, L. and Rich, T. (2002) 'E-learning and educational diversity', *Nurse Education Today*, 22 (1): 76–84.
Glen, S. and Cox, H. (2006) 'E-learning in nursing: the context', in S. Glen and P. Moule (eds), *E-learning in Nursing*. Basingstoke: Palgrave Macmillan. pp. 1–19.
Horton, W. (2000) *Designing Web-Based Training*. New York: John Wiley and Sons Inc.
Leitch, S. (2006) *Leitch Review of Skills. Prosperity for all in the global economy – world class skills. Final Report*. Retrieved from HM Treasury website: www.hm-treasury.gov.uk/media/6/4/leitch_finalreport051206.pdf

Lewis, R. and Whitlock, Q. (2003) *How to Plan and Manage an E-Learning Programme.* Aldershot: Gower.

Mason, C. and Viner, R. (2007) *E-learning Background Document: AHP in Allied Health Professionals.* London: Department of Health.

McCarthy, J. and Holt, M. (2007) 'Complexities of a policy-driven pre-registration nursing curricula', *Nursing Standard*, 22 (10): 35–8.

Moule, P. (2006) 'E-communities', in S. Glen and P. Moule (eds), *E-learning in Nursing.* Basingstoke: Palgrave Macmillan. pp. 38–53.

Pausch, R. (2002) 'A curmudgeon's vision for technology in education', in *2020 Visions Transforming Education and Training through Advanced Technologies.* Washington, DC: US Department of Commerce.

Siegel, M.A. (2002) 'The future of education', in A. Zolli (ed.), *TechTV's Catalog of Tomorrow: Trends Shaping Your Future.* Indiana: Que.

12 experiential and work-based learning

Andrea McLaughlin

DEFINITION

Experiential learning was first described by Dewey (1933), who focused on the acquisition of skills, but this has been expanded further by other educationalists and firmly liked with andragogy and learning from life (Boud et al.,1995; Burnard, 1992; Rogers, 1983). Experience is a fundamental element within many reflective models (Boud et al.,1995; Johns, 1998; Kolb, 1984) which require deconstruction and analysis of experiences, with development occurring through logical thinking, insight, reasoning, and analysis culminating in a change in behaviour. Weil and McGill (1989) proposed that experiential learning is used in four distinct areas: for gaining academic credit for work in practice; as a major learning strategy for adults; for aiding social and political change and for personal growth and development. Their ideas remain relevant and experiential learning is still utilised within these areas, particularly to help bridge the theory–practice divide.

Work-based learning is becoming increasingly important, particularly within health-related professions. It is a method of assisting students to develop by focusing on the knowledge and skills they use in their work and formulating learning objectives that are achieved within the workplace (Brennan and Little, 2006).

KEY POINTS

- Experience is fundamental to reflecting on practice.
- Experience has to be deconstructed, analysed and explored for learning to occur.
- Experience can be used to gain academic credits.

DISCUSSION

Experiential learning

Using experiential learning for teaching skills is commonplace, particularly in healthcare. The student sees a demonstration, practises the skill in a safe environment and then uses it in practice. This can build confidence, especially for skills which the student may only encounter occasionally in practice, such as resuscitation. Initially, basic or simple skills such as handwashing are experienced, with more complex skills pertinent to the profession developed later (Freeth and Fry, 2005).

Effective experiential learning should be inherent within education, introduced to students at the outset and developed to become a focal point of the learning experience. The experiential learning must be within the scope and understanding of the student, otherwise frustration may ensue and learning will not occur. To increase the students' knowledge, scenarios and problems may be used. Initially these should be simple, with more detailed scenarios subsequently employed. Problem-based learning may be done individually or with small groups, and may encompass the development of knowledge, skills and attitudes. Acquiring attributes such as attitudes and values through experiential learning can be challenging, as the individual has attitudes formed through his or her life experiences. While scenarios can be used in this respect, the main strategies are role-plays and games that require careful consideration, as these activities could be considered childish and it is important that students are able to maintain their dignity.

The benefits of experiential learning for students include taking responsibility for their own learning and developing a lifelong learning culture. Confidence, respect, empathy, trust, motivation, teamwork, autonomy, diversity, insight into the roles of others and accountability were among the major benefits identified by students in a local study in the United Kingdom (McLaughlin, 1995). Students learn about managing real problems, developing skills and coping with emotions and attitudes. Problem solving skills are transferable into practice, so students can provide logical, sound plans of care for clients. Real experiences can be discussed and the lecturer can use this to link theory to practice. Action plans for student development can be formulated, with the teacher using questions to explore the students' experiences and move learning forwards. The perceptions drawn from experience may be unique to the learner, but with guidance students can reflect on their knowledge, skills and attitudes, and so apply the learning to new situations (Rolfe, 2002).

There are challenges associated with the use of experiential learning. The lecturer needs to be adequately prepared to teach experientially, and should have the ability and expertise to intervene and prompt questions (Fowler, 2008). Lack of confidence in using experiential learning can prevent its use (McLaughlin, 1995). The lecturer and the student need to work in partnership, and self awareness and responsiveness in those in the teaching role are key factors, together with trust and empathy, as the student may reveal personal feelings, making them extremely vulnerable. Apparently trivial issues for the lecturer may be profoundly important to the student, so it is imperative that the student does not fear sarcasm and flippancy. Brackenreg (2004) sees positive facilitation of experiential learning as crucial, which, if not managed appropriately, may lead to poor learning and possibly emotional damage to the student. The lecturer's role is to help identify positive aspects of the experience, and to work through negative aspects with a non-judgemental approach.

Experiential learning in the classroom can be time-consuming with sessions taking longer to deliver and prepare than a standard lecture or seminar. As sessions often include discussion, it may be a challenge to maintain a focus. Students may diversify, if there is an urgent issue to discuss, which may require flexible management. Lecturers may find this challenging; they need therefore to be confident in the knowledge of their subject so that students derive the maximum benefit from the session.

Some students are reluctant to participate because they do not like role-play or they do not wish to share their experiences. Games and role-play can be seen as trivial (Burnard, 1992), so clear objectives are required so the student can see the context of the session. Some students may fear criticism or judgement, feel insecure or self conscious and may actively resist taking part (Fowler, 2008). Students should be made aware in advance if exploration of potentially sensitive issues is planned, so that any areas of concern can be raised prior to the session. Ground rules must be set and referred to during all experiential sessions – students must feel supported and know that confidentiality will be maintained, if they are to be honest about their feelings and actions. It is helpful to conclude experiential sessions with a discussion on the learning that has occurred.

Work-based Learning and Accreditation of Prior Experiential Learning (APEL)

Work-based learning can provide benefits for the employer, the employee and the service user. If the employer needs to develop staff to perform a specific role, then modules can be 'tailor-made' to meet those needs, for example, carrying out procedures traditionally undertaken by medical staff. Modules are developed in partnership with the Higher Education Institution (HEI) and the practice area, with joint responsibility for teaching and assessing the students who are taught in practice. This results in a practitioner who has been educated specifically, and who has been assessed as competent, in the skills required by the practice area. Service users should benefit from a better, more efficient service. Further advantages are that work-based modules are often less costly and the student does not have to be released to attend modular sessions every week (Birch et al., 2005).

Students may use experiential learning and work-based learning to claim academic credits which can then be counted towards an academic award such as a certificate, diploma or degree. Each HEI will have its own APEL processes and guidelines which will indicate which programmes permit APEL, and the amount of APEL credits that can count towards an award. For example, a student may be able to claim 50% of the required credits for an award through APEL. A typical claim is comprised of a portfolio of evidence, mapped against the relevant learning outcomes to show how the outcomes have been achieved. Portfolios may include an annotated job description, evidence of study and reflections on practice. APEL may be used within some elements of pre-qualifying programmes, but has a greater uptake by those who are already qualified and who are returning to study (Birch et al., 2005). The attraction for employers is that it provides opportunities for the staff to achieve degree-level study that is totally applied to practice.

CASE STUDY

During the first week of a pre-registration programme some student midwives identified that one of their fears was the requirement to physically examine clients, as most did not have any prior experience of this. To enable the students to experience direct physical contact, one of the lecturers who had completed a course in aromatherapy planned and delivered a session on the topic. Aromatherapy was outlined briefly, with emphasis on the fact that the students were not allowed to administer this therapy in clinical practice – the session was for information and interest only. Students then mixed their own massage oil. Working in pairs, the students massaged each other's hands with the oils, giving them the opportunity to touch another person without any threat whilst explaining exactly what they were doing to their partner. Students were asked how they felt when they were massaged; how it felt to give the massage; whether explaining the procedure helped or not; and what the positive and negative aspects of the experience were. The session was evaluated well.

CONCLUSION

Experiential learning can assist students to gain knowledge as they experience 'finding out' and ascertaining the knowledge they need to aid them in decision making processes. It can help with skills acquisition, allowing the student to practise in a safe environment. Formation and development of attitudes and values may be linked with an increase in knowledge and skills and also from the use of role-play and debate. For some, using APEL, and work-based learning, may provide opportunities to gain further qualifications.

Learning derived from experience is traditionally not seen to be as scientific or as relevant as learning from research evidence, however it has been shown to be of exceptional value to the student (Rolfe, 2002). Therefore, if the aim is to develop the student, then experiential learning is inherent within the role of the teacher.

See also: academic staff development; clinical competence; practice teaching; problem-based learning; reflection; simulated learning and OSCEs; teaching strategies

FURTHER READING

Fowler, J. (2008) 'Experiential learning and its facilitation', *Nurse Education Today*, 28 (4): 427–33.

REFERENCES

Birch, L., McLaughlin, A. and Somerville, D. (2005) 'Work-based studies: one small step for the individual, a giant leap for the NHS', *British Journal of Midwifery*, 13 (11): 727–31.

Boud, D., Keogh, R. and Walker, D. (eds) (1995) *Turning Reflection into Learning.* London: Kogan Page.

Brackenreg, J. (2004) 'Issues in reflection and debriefing: how nurse education structures experiential activities', *Nurse Education in Practice*, 4 (4): 264–70.

Brennan, J. and Little, B. (2006) *Towards a Strategy for Workplace Learning: Report of a Study to Assist HEFCE in the Development of a Strategy for Workplace Learning.* London: Centre for Higher Education, Research and Information.

Burnard, P. (1992) 'Defining experiential learning: nurse tutors' perceptions', *Nurse Education Today*, 12 (1): 29–36.

Dewey, J. (1933) *How We Think.* Boston, MA: Heath.

Fowler, J. (2008) 'Experiential learning and its facilitation', *Nurse Education Today*, 28 (4): 427–33.

Freeth, D. and Fry, H. (2005) 'Nursing students' and tutors' perceptions of learning and teaching in a clinical skills centre', *Nurse Education Today*, 25 (4): 272–82.

Johns, C. (1998) 'Opening the doors of perception', in C. Johns and D. Freshwater (eds), *Transforming Nursing through Reflective Practice.* London: Blackwell Science. pp. 1–20.

Kolb, D. (1984) *Experiential Learning: Experience as the Source of Learning.* Englewood Cliffs, NJ: Prentice-Hall.

McLaughlin, A. (1995) 'Attitudes to Experiential Learning in a School of Midwifery', University of Liverpool: Unpublished MEd dissertation.

Rogers, C.R. (1983) *Freedom to Learn for the 80s.* London: Merrill.

Rolfe, G. (2002) 'Reflective practice; where now?', *Nurse Education in Practice*, 2 (1): 21–9.

Weil, S.W. and McGill, I. (1989) *Making Sense of Experiential Learning.* Milton Keynes: Open University Press.

13 feedback and marking

Annette McIntosh

DEFINITION

Feedback has several general meanings, but in the academic context it can be defined as the giving of advice pertaining to an individual's performance, from which the recipient may improve and develop through having a clearer understanding of the expected standards (Fry et al., 2009). It is widely agreed that feedback is central to effective student learning, although as Carless (2006) noted, the process involved is more complex than is often realised or acknowledged.

Marking is the provision of a mark or grade to establish the standard of achievement of a student's performance (Quality Assurance Agency (QAA), 2006), involving consideration of many elements in order to ensure the quality of the process.

KEY POINTS

- The provision of quality feedback is central to the progress and development of students, and there are core principles that can guide all staff involved in the process.
- Ensuring the quality of marking assessments is a key consideration for Higher Education Institutions (HEIs), necessitating the development and operation of regulations and principles to guide markers.

DISCUSSION

Feedback

Providing feedback to students is a central tenet of ensuring and enhancing the quality of learning. This entails (HEIs) operating processes that offer feedback to students in such a way that learning and improvement is facilitated, whilst not increasing the overall assessment load (QAA, 2006). The essential role of feedback has been further highlighted by the United Kingdom's National Union of Students (NUS), who state that it is evident from national surveys that students are concerned about poor assessment feedback and that this impacts negatively on their learning and development (Porter, 2009). To address these concerns, the NUS compiled ten principles for good feedback practice (Porter, 2009:1), stating that feedback should:

- be *for* learning, not just *of* learning.
- be a continuous process.
- be timely.
- relate to clear criteria.
- be constructive.
- be legible and clear.
- be provided on exams.
- include self-assessment and peer–peer feedback.
- be accessible to all students.
- be flexible and suited to students' needs.

Nicol and MacFarlane-Dick (2006) had earlier developed a model of seven core principles of good feedback practice, some of which are incorporated in the NUS framework. Additional to the NUS model are the principles of: promotion of peer and tutor dialogue around learning; provision of opportunities to close the gap between current and desired performance; delivery of high quality information to students about their learning; encouragement of positive motivational beliefs and self esteem and provision of information to teachers that may be used to help shape the teaching (Nicol and MacFarlane-Dick, 2006). The principles of both models are underpinned by a number of considerations.

Feedback can take a number of forms, including formative, summative, informal, formal, oral, written and generic and can be given on a continuous basis or at set points during a module or programme of study. A range of individuals may be involved in providing feedback depending on the assessment task, from academic staff and peers for theory-based assignments to practitioners and service users for clinical or performance-based components.

The provision of feedback needs to be a planned element in the assessment process, with both staff and students being clear about the type, purpose and timing of the feedback. Weaver (2006) researched students' perceptions of written feedback and reported four main themes that were seen as unhelpful: feedback that was too general or vague; feedback that lacked guidance; negatively focused comments and feedback not related to the assessment criteria. Clearly, ensuring the quality of the feedback process is important. In the UK, the QAA set out standards of good practice and operational elements in an assessment code of practice, offering guidance for all those involved in designing and giving feedback (QAA, 2006).

Whilst it is widely agreed that feedback is central to the learning process, with many considerations to address in ensuring the quality of feedback, inherent in the whole process is the premise that students use and value feedback to reflect on, and enhance, their work. Researchers in the field report this as a relatively unexplored area (Carless, 2006; Weaver, 2006), although various recent studies have addressed the student viewpoint. Carless (2006) reported that the students in his study had differing perspectives to staff on some elements of the feedback process, with lecturers believing the feedback they provided was more detailed and useful feedback than the students did and the perception of some lecturing staff that students' interest lay solely in their awarded grades was not borne out. Weaver (2006) showed that whilst students reported that they valued feedback, it was evident that some may require guidance and help in understanding and acting upon the feedback, before fully engaging with it. Yorke (2003) considered that awareness of the psychological elements involved in the giving and receiving of feedback was of vital importance to the process, alongside the content of the feedback.

It is evident that the feedback process is multi-faceted and complex and, as the QAA (2006) noted, HEIs must ensure staff development in this process, as well as in the equally important concept of marking.

Marking

There is a plethora of assessment methods used within professional programmes, including those carried out in practice, testing not only the theoretical knowledge of students, but also their skills and attitudes. Current initiatives in professional education include the grading of practice which brings with it particular challenges of designing appropriate tools and marking criteria.

All HEIs are required to have robust mechanisms in place to ensure the quality of the marking processes pertaining to all types of assessment and it is important that this is considered in the planning stages of a programme or module. There are commonly agreed basic principles associated with marking. In essence, the process should be:

- consistent and fair – as the QAA (2006) notes, HEIs have a responsibility to ensure and achieve consistency across the institution, not only in grading work, but also when considering such elements as extenuating, or mitigating, circumstances.
- valid, in that the marking measures that which it sets out to measure, including the level of taxonomy.
- reliable – as Norton (2009) considers, this is usually achieved through the use of marking criteria or schemes, helping different markers to grade work comparably.
- transparent and explicit, where all elements of the marking process are clear, unambiguous and communicated in an open and timely manner to all concerned in the process, especially students.
- able to demonstrate rigour, probity and security (QAA, 2006).
- inclusive, ensuring that reasonable adjustments are made for students with disabilities such as dyslexia or hearing difficulties (Norton, 2009).

Upholding the above principles requires HEIs to ensure that their assessment regulations are adhered to and that all staff have a clear understanding of, and are competent to undertake, their responsibilities in this respect (QAA, 2006). Marking processes can include anonymous marking, where applicable, and should involve internal verification measures such as second or double marking. A moderation system also has to be in place, involving both internal and external examiners. This helps to provide assurance that the marking criteria have been consistently applied and that the final assessment outcomes are both reliable and fair (QAA, 2006). Another factor becoming increasingly important is that of plagiarism and many HEIs are taking active steps to detect and reduce the incidence by using plagiarism detection software systems, alongside the use of policies to deter the practice and guide and advise students on what constitutes plagiarism.

However, whilst all these processes help evidence the aim of academics to be seen to be objective and fair in their marking, as Norton (2009) pointed out, it is well known that students are less convinced of the consistency of marking, and this view may be well founded. Carless (2006) showed that while lecturers believed that their marking was fair, students had much more mixed feelings about the fairness of the grading of assessments. Norton (2009) noted that in the wealth of research on assessment, many studies highlight the difficulties involved in assuring the quality of the processes; this again highlights the imperative for staff development, assistance and support in order for lecturers to have confidence and competence in all elements of marking.

CASE STUDY

A team of lecturers delivers the same undergraduate module to large cohorts of students across three different sites. In order to ensure the rigour and fairness of marking the summative essay element, the team uses level-related criteria and a marking scheme with expected content to guide team members' grading of the scripts. One lecturer, new to the team and to marking, is mentored by an experienced academic. The assignments are not double-marked, as it is the HEI's policy only to do so in relation to the dissertation module at undergraduate level. Internal moderation of a sample of the scripts, including all fails, borderline passes and scripts from all other grading bands, is carried out by an allocated lecturer from outwith the module team. The moderator's report is included with the sample sent to the external examiner.

The internal and external moderation processes uphold the marks awarded and the reports indicate that due process was followed, a representative spread of marks was evident and that the grading was fair and consistent across sites. However, it is noted in both the internal and external moderation reports that the quality of feedback to students was variable. In particular, some was very brief, vague and handwritten, which was hard to read, whilst other lecturers had given very full, specific and word-processed feedback. Some of the team had annotated comments in the scripts, whilst others had not.

These comments were noted, along with other similar comments from moderators of other modules, by the faculty. In order to address the issue, further staff development days on the assessment process were run, covering the principles of good practice in feedback and including a session with student representatives. A subsequent improvement in the quality of feedback to students was noted and commented on positively in internal and external reports.

CONCLUSION

The concepts of feedback and marking are important elements in the education process and there are many considerations for all involved. In order for students to progress and develop, there are basic principles for good practice in feedback. In relation to marking, the quality of processes is paramount, guided by regulations and adherence to the basic principles of assessment practice. Staff development and support are key factors in assuring the quality of both feedback and marking.

See also: academic staff development; assessment; dealing with failing and problem students; quality assurance and enhancement

FURTHER READING

Quality Assurance Agency (2006) The *Code of Practice for the Assurance of Academic Quality and Standards in Higher Education, Section 6 – Assessment of Students*, 2nd edn. Mansfield: Linney Direct.

REFERENCES

Carless, D. (2006) 'Differing perceptions in the feedback process', *Studies in Higher Education*, 31 (2): 219–33.

Fry, H., Ketteridge, S. and Marshall, S. (2009) *A Handbook for Teaching and Learning in Higher Education*, 3rd edn. London: Routledge.

Nicol, D.J. and MacFarlane-Dick, D. (2006) 'Formative assessment and self regulated learning: a model and 7 principles of good feedback', *Studies in Higher Education*, 31 (2): 199–218.

Norton, L. (2009) 'Assessing student learning', in H. Fry, S. Ketteridge and A. Marshall (eds), *A Handbook for Teaching and Learning in Higher Education*, 3rd edn. London: Routledge. pp 132–49.

Porter, A. (2009) 'NUS – working to improve assessment feedback', *HE Focus*, 1: 1.

Quality Assurance Agency (2006) *The Code of Practice for the Assurance of Academic Quality and Standards in Higher Education, Section 6 – Assessment of Students*, 2nd edn. Mansfield: Linney Direct.

Weaver, M.R. (2006) 'Do students value feedback? Student perceptions of tutors' written responses', *Assessment and Evaluation in Higher Education*, 31 (3): 379–94.

Yorke, M. (2003) 'Formative assessment in higher education: moves towards theory and the enhancement of pedagogic practice', *Higher Education*, 45 (4): 477–501.

feedback and marking

14 humanist learning theories

Annette McIntosh

DEFINITION

Humanist learning theories derive from the philosophical stance of phenomenology, being essentially concerned with the feelings, thoughts, values and experiences of individuals in relation to their growth and fulfilment. The education of healthcare professionals is seen to be broadly dominated by educational theories deriving from the humanistic perspective, especially given the paradigm shift in recent years from preparing professionals using training courses to situating programmes with Higher Education (Purdy, 1997a). Key influences in this respect were Bevis and Watson (1989), who argued for a shift from the behavioural paradigm used to underpin nursing programmes, to a curriculum model based on humanist and caring principles.

KEY POINTS

- Humanist learning theories concern the individual and his or her thoughts, feelings and motivations.
- Learning approaches include experiential learning and andragogy, with educators adopting a facilitative role.
- Criticisms include a lack of evidence base to substantiate the approach and the lack of acknowledgement of social and cultural influences on education.
- In the healthcare professions, the use of humanistically derived learning theories is widespread, and though often challenging, it can be seen to have benefits for students and the professions.

DISCUSSION

Learning theories deriving from the humanist ideology differ from others in that they embrace the affective domain of learning and are based on the assumption that all individuals are unique and are motivated to grow in a positive way. As Braungart and Braungart (2008) noted, the humanistic perspective purports that the feelings and emotions of an individual are key elements in the learning process and that the primary goals for educators are encouraging and stimulating the curiosity, initiative, interest and sense of responsibility of learners.

The work of John Dewey in the early 1900s is seen to be the base from which the humanist philosophy of learning grew, with Gregory (2006) stating that Dewey's thinking on progressive education influenced, and continues to influence, educators of the humanistic persuasion. These include Maslow, Rogers and Knowles, as discussed below.

Maslow (1971) espoused a theory of motivation and a hierarchical ordering of needs: a basic level of physiological needs followed by safety needs, the need to belong, the need for self esteem, and, at the highest level, the need for self actualisation and the fulfilment of potential. Maslow considered that the lower level of needs had to be at least partially fulfilled in order for an individual to ascend to the next higher order of needs. Consequently, the goal for educators is facilitate learners to achieve self actualisation and reach their maximum potential. Critics note that there is little in the way of research to uphold Maslow's theory, and that higher-level activities such as learning and self fulfilment may be achieved by those who have not met their basic levels of needs (Braungart and Braungart, 2008).

Carl Rogers, a psychotherapist by background, developed the notion of student-centred learning from his approach of client-centred therapy, which involved the constructive development, including self awareness, of the individual through a process involving a facilitator. Rogers (1983) considered that these principles could be transferred to the learning process and identified a learning continuum with meaningless material at one end and meaningful material at the other: the meaningless material held no relevance for the individual and did not involve feelings, while the meaningful, experiential material concerned both thoughts and feelings and was significant to the individual. Rogers (1983) set out five elements for significant experiential learning: involvement of the whole person; self initiation; pervasiveness; evaluation by the student and finally, that the essence of the learning is meaningful. The implications of these principles for those in teaching roles include valuing and trusting students, placing them at the centre of the experience and, essentially, giving students freedom to learn.

Knowles, in developing a theoretical framework for adult learning in the 1960s, adopted the term andragogy, coined by educators in Europe, and defined as 'the art and science of helping adults learn' (Knowles, 1984: 6). Knowles declared that andragogy might not be considered a theory *per se*, but more a system of concepts. He states that the assumptions of andragogy include the following:

- The learner is self directing, based on the premise that adults need to take responsibility for themselves and can resent or resist being treated like children.
- Adults enter into education with a different volume and quality of experience and are therefore the richest resources for each other. Methods such

as group discussion, problem-based learning and learning plans and contracts make use of this experience.

- Adults become ready to learn when they perceive a need to know or develop skills in an aspect of their lives.
- The orientation to learning is life-centred, task-centred or problem-centred.
- The motivation to learn is underpinned predominantly by internal factors such as self esteem, recognition and self actualisation.

In addition, Knowles (1984) proposed seven elements in the design and implementation of an andragogical approach in programmes of education:

- setting the appropriate climate for learning, including ensuring an appropriate physical climate and engendering a conducive psychological climate (the latter involves elements such as mutual respect and trust, collaboration, support, openness and what Knowles termed a climate of humanness).
- involving students in a mutual planning process.
- involving students in diagnosing their own learning needs.
- involving students in formulating their own learning outcomes.
- involving students in designing their own learning plans.
- helping students achieve their learning plans.
- involving students in evaluating their learning.

While it is recognised that the education of healthcare professionals is widely underpinned by tenets of the humanist tradition, there are critics of the approach. For example, Tennant (1998), in considering postmodern critiques of learning theories, opined that traditions embracing humanistic and andragogical learning approaches failed to take into account the power of social and cultural forces in education. Merriam noted that the notions of andragogy and self directed learning have been criticised for a 'blinding focus on the individual learner while ignoring the sociohistorical context in which it occurs' (2001: 11). Braungart and Braungart (2008) also stated that humanist learning theories have weaknesses, including the fact that the claimed strengths of the approach are not substantiated by research and that a particular criticism concerns the promotion of learners who are self-centred and unable to take criticism.

There are further challenges associated with the use of humanistic approaches, well expressed by Gregory, who stated that 'the idea that formal (traditional) education might concern itself with the emotional and inner life of the person remains a curious and potentially risky idea to many' (2006: 115). Braungart and Braungart (2008) also considered that the use of the humanistic stance can make some educators, and students, feel uncomfortable, due to the cult-like 'touchy feely' approach. Milligan (1997) noted that some educators were reluctant to adopt an andragogical approach to their teaching, due to their traditional views and resistance to move the power and control in the educational relationship in favour of the students.

Notwithstanding these concerns, however, it remains the case that humanistic approaches in healthcare education have real merits and are in widespread use. As Braungart and Braungart (2008) noted, approaches to education have been modified due to the central placement of the needs, feelings and values of the student in the learning process, with the concomitant redefinition of the role of the educator. Merriam (2001) stated that humanist-based approaches have become an integral part of the adult education process, with an important impact on teaching practice, whilst Burnard (1989) opined that the combined use of andragogy and experiential learning offered a powerful medium for fostering the range of expertise necessary for healthcare professionals, including clinical, intellectual, interpersonal and social skills.

There can be seen to be dissonance in the criteria-driven curricula required by the professional bodies in healthcare and the adoption of humanistic approaches to learning. Purdy (1997b) considered that the use of strategies such as self-directed learning has been shown to be problematic due to the need to meet the specific, prescribed content in educational programmes. However, as Milligan (1997) noted, in line with the thinking of Burnard (1989), the very nature of becoming, and being, a healthcare professional requires qualities that can be seen to be fostered through the use of humanistic approaches such as andragogy and experiential learning. Ultimately, given the current drivers for educating in healthcare, it can be seen that programmes may have to embrace elements of a number of learning theories to ensure the best possible experiences and outcomes for both the students and the profession. As Braungart and Braungart stated 'in practice, learning theories should not be considered to be mutually exclusive but rather to operate together to change attitudes and behaviour' (2008: 81).

CASE STUDY

A programme planning team is developing a new programme for post-registration specialist nursing. The team includes academic, clinical, service user and student representation. Prior to the first meeting, the chairperson asks the team members to come prepared with their views on the underpinning educational philosophy for the programme and how they would like to see the educational processes planned to best facilitate student learning and achievement.

At the outset of the meeting the chairperson outlined the professional and academic requirements to be met for validation, which necessitated an outcome-based curriculum approach, including clinical competences. On debating the underpinning theoretical stance for the programme, it became evident that the views of the team were largely of the humanist persuasion. The student, service user and clinical representatives were particularly keen on placing the student at the centre of their learning and adopting a very adult-focused, experiential approach to learning, which they felt reflected the holistic basis of modern healthcare. However, a few members of the academic staff were concerned about the need for the students to achieve specific, professional goals in a tight timescale and felt that a much more structured and didactic approach was called for. In the ensuing discussions, the team agreed that in order to meet the minimal requirements and boundaries of the curriculum, a mix of learning theories and strategies would be used, but that the overriding stance should be one of an andragogical, humanistically based approach to learning.

CONCLUSION

Learning theories and strategies deriving from the humanist tradition have been widely adopted in the education for, and of, the healthcare professions. While there are criticisms of the approach and many challenges for educators, both strategic and pragmatic, using humanist learning theories can be seen to have many benefits for students, placing them squarely at the centre of their learning experience.

See also: curriculum models and design; experiential and work-based learning; learning environments; peer support and observation; transformative learning

FURTHER READING

Quinn, F. and Hughes, S. (2007) 'Adult learning theory', in F. Quinn and S. Hughes (eds), *Quinn's Principles and Practice of Nurse Education*, 5th edn. Cheltenham, UK: Nelson Thornes. pp. 17–52.

REFERENCES

Bevis, E.O. and Watson, J. (1989) *Toward a Caring Curriculum: A New Pedagogy for Nursing*. New York: National League for Nursing.

Braungart M.M. and Braungart, R.G. (2008) 'Applying learning theories to healthcare practice', in S.B. Bastable (ed.), *Nurse as Educator*, 2nd edn. Sudbury, MA: Jones and Bartlett. pp. 51–84.

Burnard, P. (1989) 'Experiential learning and andragogy – negotiated learning in nurse education: a critical appraisal', *Nurse Education Today*, 9 (5): 300–6.

Gregory, J. (2006) 'Experiential learning', in P. Jarvis (ed.), *The Theory and Practice of Teaching*, 2nd edn. London: Routledge. pp. 114–29.

Knowles, M. (1984) 'Introduction: the art and science of helping adults learn', in M. Knowles and Associates *Andragogy in Action. Applying Modern Principles of Adult Learning*. San Francisco, CA: Jossey-Bass. pp. 1–24.

Maslow, A. (1971) *The Farther Reaches of Human Nature*. Harmondsworth: Penguin.

Merriam, S.B. (2001) 'Andragogy and self directed learning: pillars of adult learning theory', *New Directions for Adult and Continuing Education, No. 89*. Retrieved from www.fsu.edu/~elps/ae/download/ade5385/Merriam.pdf

Milligan, F. (1997) 'In defence of andragogy. Part 2: An educational process consistent with modern nursing's aims', *Nurse Education Today*, 17 (6): 487–93.

Purdy, M. (1997a) 'Humanist ideology and nurse education. 1. Humanist educational theory', *Nurse Education Today*, 17 (3): 192–5.

Purdy, M. (1997b) 'Humanist ideology and nurse education. 2. Limitations of humanist educational theory in nurse education', *Nurse Education Today*, 17 (3): 196–202.

Rogers, C. (1983) *Freedom to Learn for the 80s.* Colombus, OH: Merrill.

Tennant, M. (1998) 'Adult education as a technology of the self', *International Journal of Lifelong Education*, 17 (6): 364–76.

15 information literacy

Wendy Fiander

DEFINITION

The concepts and themes of information literacy are well established and of particular significance for healthcare. For educators in healthcare it is possible to embed relevant information literacy content at appropriate times during any programme. Institutional subject librarians can work collaboratively with educators to achieve this.

An authoritative definition of information literacy is from the Chartered Institute of Library and Information Professionals (CILIP): 'Information literacy is knowing when and why you need information, where to find it, and how to evaluate, use and communicate it in an ethical manner'. It follows, therefore, that:

an information literate person can understand:

- a need for information.
- availability of resources.
- how to find information.
- the need to evaluate results.
- how to work with or exploit results.
- ethics and responsibility of use.
- how to communicate or share their findings.
- how to manage their findings.

(CILIP, 2004)

A wider concept is that of 'digital literacy', where an individual is 'capable of handling information and mediating their interactions with social and professional groups using an ever-changing and expanding range of digital technologies' (Francis and Burholt, 2009). These skills should then be placed within the context of evidence-based medicine or care, where individual clinical expertise is integrated with the best available evidence from systematic research when making treatment decisions (Sackett, 2000). It follows that an ability to identify and use the highest available quality of information is critical to a high standard of work during health-care education and excellent quality of healthcare during a subsequent career.

KEY POINTS

- Information literacy is particularly important to healthcare students.
- Information literacy comprises a range of skills relating to the retrieval and management of knowledge.
- Information literacy is becoming increasingly important as global technology develops.
- Collaboration between information professionals and academic staff is vital for the effective learning of these skills.

DISCUSSION

A useful model for outlining the themes and levels within the concept of information literacy was developed by the United Kingdom Society of National University and College Libraries (SCONUL, 2004). Implicit within the model are two strands in the acquisition of information literacy skills. Firstly there are competences generally related to 'study skills', including the ability to use an institutional library and to retrieve and cite literature as necessary. Then there are competences beyond this, still required after formal education. These include an understanding of the origins, management, dissemination and exploitation of information; the ability to critically appraise the content and validity of any information; and an ability to embrace new and constantly developing digital technologies and use them effectively in a social and professional context.

The model encompasses seven headline skills (portrayed diagrammatically in Figure 15.1 as pillars), with examples of the specific activity or competency that illustrates the application of each skill:

1. the ability to recognise a need for information.
2. the ability to distinguish ways in which the information 'gap' may be addressed.
3. the ability to construct strategies for locating information.
4. the ability to locate and access information.
5. the ability to compare and evaluate information obtained from different sources.

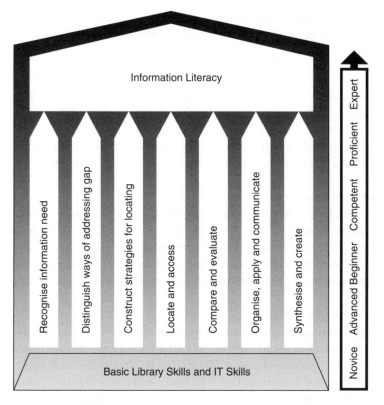

Figure 15.1 The SCONUL seven pillars model for information literacy (reprinted with permission from SCONUL)

6. the ability to organise, apply and communicate information to others in ways appropriate to the situation.
7. the ability to synthesise and build upon existing information, contributing to the creation of new knowledge.

(SCONUL, 2004)

The SCONUL model recognises the fundamental foundation of basic library and IT skills to support the acquisition of the seven information skills 'pillars'. By adding the dimension showing progression from 'novice' to 'expert' for each skill, the model recognises the need to progress from the first level of 'education'-related competence to the greater expertise required for a fully 'information literate' person. First-year undergraduates would usually be categorised as 'novice' to 'advanced beginner', perhaps only practising the first four skills, while postgraduate and research students would be working at the 'expert' end of the scale and practising all seven skills.

The educator and information professional can together develop learning outcomes and subject content to map onto these skills at progressive levels of competence. Some of the concepts that can be included in the content of information skills or literacy sessions are as follows.

The 'structure' of academic literature

It is helpful to describe the different categories of publication in which knowledge may appear as it is developed and used by different authors, including the 'invisible college' and primary or secondary literature. With an understanding of this publication process and structure, students can select appropriate categories to search for their research requirements.

Systematic searching

Techniques for phrasing and analysing questions to search most efficiently for information include the use of concepts, keywords and synonyms, an understanding of particular methods for combining terms systematically and an appreciation of the value of using controlled vocabularies and other imposed indexing systems for the effective retrieval of information.

Role of the Internet

The Internet makes high quality information more accessible and at the same time more challenging to retrieve. It is vital for students to understand how information is published on the Internet, to be able to find and select trustworthy sites, and to have skills for critically evaluating the information they retrieve. Students today can be described as the 'Google generation' (Centre for Information Behaviour and the Evaluation of Research, 2008) and exhibit different information processing skills than previous generations. For them it is important to reinforce the methods of effective searching for high quality academic information, some of which may be provided only by their university or Trust (the 'deep' Web) rather than via popular search engines (the 'surface' Web).

Critical appraisal

The skills necessary to evaluate retrieved information are particularly important when working within the context of evidence-based healthcare. Gray (2007) stated: 'Professionals and patients need clean clear knowledge for decision making just as they need clean clear water for hand washing. Water may look clear but be polluted and poisonous.' Critical appraisal is necessary for all information, printed or electronic, and with the increased sharing of content via the Internet this skill is more significant. Several methodologies can be taught and assessed within a research methods module, or included within information skills sessions.

Responsible use and communication of information

There are options for the management of the documents and information that students discover. The concept of plagiarism is increasingly topical and requires exploration, combined with a full explanation about correct referencing. Examples at the competent/expert level are the skills of synthesis and analysis required for the production of an academic literature review.

Edwards and Bruce (2002) use common metaphors to describe an increase in the range of skills for ineffective information retrieval:

- for a novice, the problem is equivalent to 'finding a needle in a haystack';
- for a more information literate person with limited knowledge and tools, finding information is viewed as 'working through a maze';
- those with the highest levels of competency and knowledge about the information environment are able to 'pan for gold' and to effectively retrieve only the high-quality 'nuggets' of information.

Whilst information literacy was an important concept before the availability of electronic information resources, it is of much greater significance for successful employment, citizenship and lifelong learning now that so much information is published electronically. The range in information quality available and in methods of access requires additional knowledge and skills for effective retrieval.

Online and independent learning developments increase further the need to ensure that students can support their learning by accessing high-quality information sources. The development of digital literacy is central to any institutional strategy for increasing technology-enhanced learning.

Some of the reasons for the importance of these skills are:

- People are searching for information in greater quantity and using it with increased impact.
- The information environment is much more chaotic and less controlled, resulting in significant problems about quality.
- People may be working more in isolation, with little support for effective retrieval.
- On the Web the derivation of the information presented may be masked from the user – a 'black box' approach. Tools for retrieval are often simplified for the user, so hiding complexities and reducing options.
- Users may be satisfied by obtaining information that is 'good enough' when they are not fully aware of the full range of sources available and effective methods of retrieval.
- Students are learning in a different way and are much more willing to share knowledge and information, often using Web 2.0 facilities such as blogs.

It is also important to recognise that the 'information environment' available to people will differ depending on their status. For example, the significant academic resources accessible to university students will depend on the purchasing policy of their library and may differ from those available to qualified healthcare professionals via their employing organisation. The access arrangements to physical collections and the licences governing the rights to use electronic resources significantly restrict universal access to resources by all who might want to use them. For students in healthcare, therefore, it is important to offer guidance about the different information environment they will experience when employed, so that they can use it effectively without delay.

Effective liaison between the healthcare educator and the information professionals in the institution library service is a key factor in the successful embedding of information literacy content in the curriculum with the delivery of timely, relevant and interesting content. The library staff will usually be keen and competent to work with faculty members to achieve a key objective of increasing student information literacy.

If librarians are included at the planning stage of a new programme they can find opportunities to match other needs of the curriculum with the information literacy agenda. Such professionals are aware of emerging technologies in the information environment and can suggest ways to incorporate them into educational programmes. When the programme is delivered these staff can do far more than provide solely an introduction to the library resources, by delivering content at points of most relevance and need over the duration of the programme. This may be in the context of problem-based learning, when the librarian can introduce key sources, or help to prepare for assignments, where information about search techniques or referencing can be delivered. The explicit collaboration between educator and librarian at these points can improve the motivation and attentiveness of students and result in work of a higher quality.

CASE STUDY

At the University of Chester in the UK, learning outcomes based on the SCONUL seven pillar model are used by librarians for a series of information skills sessions throughout the healthcare programmes, as follows:

- At induction, students are introduced to the mechanics of the University of Chester network, virtual learning environment and library catalogue, in line with the 'novice/beginner' level of the model.
- A further session includes the formulation of simple information search strategies, use of full text journal collections and effective searching of the Internet, mapping onto the 'advanced beginner' level of the model.
- Referencing and related concepts are introduced by academic staff at the same time.
- An assessed assignment tests these fundamental skills and reinforces their importance.
- Skill levels are then increased at strategic points throughout the programme. Bibliographic databases are introduced at the end of the first year, supported by revision of search strategy techniques. A session before leaving the programme prepares students for the different information environment they will encounter outside of university.

CONCLUSION

Teaching a wide range of information literacy skills during a healthcare education programme will provide significant support to a high quality of education and to excellent professional healthcare. Developing technologies require that skills evolve and that students are provided with effective tools to retrieve and manage reputable information. Through close liaison between information professionals and healthcare educators during the programme, students can acquire these skills at different levels at points when they are most relevant to their needs.

See also: curriculum planning and development; E-learning; problem-based learning; research and scholarly activity; study skills

FURTHER READING

Information Literacy (2009) Retrieved from Information Literacy website: www.information literacy.org.uk

Rumsey, S. (2008) *How to Find Information: A Guide for Researchers.* Maidenhead: Open University Press.

REFERENCES

Centre for Information Behaviour and the Evaluation of Research (2008) *Information Behaviour of the Researcher of the Future: A CIBER Briefing Paper.* London: University College London.

CILIP (Chartered Institute of Library and Information Professionals) (2004) *Information Literacy.* Retrieved from CILIP website: www.cilip.org.uk

Edwards, S.L. and Bruce, C.S. (2002) 'Needles, Haystacks, Filters and Me: The IT Confidence Dilemma', in *Lifelong Learning Conference: Refereed Papers from the 2nd International Lifelong Learning Conference.* Yeppoon, Central Queensland, Australia, 16–19 June 2002. pp. 165–71.

Francis, R. and Burholt, S. (2009) *Developing Digital Literacies in a Wiki Environment.* Retrieved from Oxford Brookes University website: www.brookes.ac.uk/download/ attachments/1900727/shock_poster_0409.pdf?version=1

Gray, M. (2007) Key note presentation at LILAC (Librarians Information Literacy Annual Conference) 2007. Retrieved from CILIP website: www.cilip.org.uk/specialinterest-groups/bysubject/informationliteracy/lilac/lilac2007

Sackett, D (2000) *Evidence-based Medicine: How to Practise and Teach EBM,* 2nd edn. London: Churchill Livingstone.

SCONUL Advisory Committee on Information Literacy (2004) *Information Skills in Higher Education: Briefing Paper.* Retrieved from SCONUL website: www.sconul.ac.uk/groups/ information_literacy/papers/Seven_pillars2.pdf

16 interprofessional learning

Aidan Worsley

DEFINITION

The United Kingdom Centre for the Advancement of Interprofessional Education defines interprofessional learning (IPL) as 'the occasions when two or more professions learn from and about each other to improve collaboration and the quality of care' (Walsh et al., 2005: 231). This can be differentiated from *multi*-professional learning which denotes more of a simpler 'shared' form of learning by two or more professions who happen to be learning together. *Inter*professional learning is a more purposeful, focused attempt to learn together to make a difference. As Barr, one of the major influences in this field stated, IPL concerns:

> the application of principles of adult learning to interactive, group-based learning, which relates collaborative learning to collaborative practice within a coherent rationale and which is informed by an understanding of interpersonal, group, inter-group, organisational and inter-organisational relations and processes of professionalisation. (2002: 23)

KEY POINTS

- The evidence base for IPL is still emerging.
- The complexity of IPL and its situated nature suggest that localised solutions might be best.
- Professional identity is intertwined with IPL and transformational learning experiences are likely to involve deep personal reflection.
- Learner-centred, situated, positive social learning based on authentic problems forms the basis of a way forward.
- Educators should ensure that IPL is carefully evaluated.

DISCUSSION

It is hard to separate the drivers for interprofessional education from those for interprofessional working. If we consider developments in government policy and general health and social care practice over the past decade or so, the push for 'joined up' thinking and working is evident, and has been responded to within the educational frameworks surrounding qualifying and post-qualifying professional programmes (Dutton and Worsley, 2009). One illustration would be the succession of UK public inquiries, such as the Victoria Climbié Inquiry (Laming, 2003). The central theme remains the same: inquiries underline the importance of professions working together, yet find that they don't. The notion of professional 'tribes' appears stronger than teams of people (Mead, 2007). Most recently in the UK, the inquiry into the death of 'Baby P' and the actions of health bodies (other inquiries considered police and social care workers), conducted by the Care Quality Commission revealed a scenario of staff shortages, poor training and inadequate communication as National Health Service staff missed 35 opportunities to identify and protect the child at risk. The report identified a number of systematic failings of which it notes first, 'Poor communication between health professionals and between agencies, leading to a lack of urgent action with regard to child protection arrangements, and no effective escalation of concern' (Care Quality Commission, 2009: 36).

It is clear from such documents and policy directives that both evidence and a strong perception exist that support a view that insufficient attention is being paid to interprofessional working.

In a similar vein we can see the exhortations of policy drivers to deliver on IPL but a frustratingly limited body of evidence that shows how to do it well. Documents from a health-based perspective that are indicative of the drivers of central policy development with regard to interprofessional education include a *Health Service of All Talents* (Department of Health (DH), 2000) which specifically requires that pre-qualifying programmes for nurses include an element of preparation for interprofessional practice. Pollard et al. (2004) subsequently looked at a large group of nursing and social work qualifying students in Bristol, UK. In a nutshell, one of their core findings was that both professional groups were clearly positive about IPL, thinking it was a good idea. However, both groups were far less positive about the prospect of interaction between these groups. They didn't wish to learn together about working together. Effective IPL is, according to Salmon and Jones (2001: 19), a 'nebulous phenomenon' – a search for which is likened to that for the 'holy grail' (Mattick and Bligh, 2006: 399). Mead (2007) talks of the series of false starts and false dawns of IPL. He highlights disappointment and disillusion with the post-2000 interprofessional education agenda, observing its movement from a central to a secondary concern and suggests that in some policy documents, such as the White Paper *Our Health, Our Care, Our Say* (DH, 2006), the concept appears to have disappeared altogether. Barr et al. (2005) argue that the evidence is growing in stature and comprehensiveness.

So, what appears to have soured the IPL dream? Some authors critique the notion of joined up working as both simplistic and conservative. They argue that the ideology underpinning this notion rests upon an assumption that different professional groups are content to work with each other in a peaceful and ultimately benevolent manner within a shared value base. Transparently, this is not the case. Furthermore, they assert that the construction of multi-disciplinary working as an answer to the most complex problems of service delivery leads to inward-looking explorations of resources and constant reorganisation at the expense of more imaginative, localised, community-based responses to client need (Easen et al., 2000). Anning (2005) takes this idea a step further and suggests that it is naïve to imagine the complex demands of policy around interprofessional working can be met with simple, global exhortations to 'join up'; what is required is a greater emphasis on researching the effectiveness of these emerging new team shapes and structures as they respond to this emerging complexity.

It is vitally important that the acceptance of IPL as a problematic concept should not lead to its rejection. To a greater or lesser extent practitioners and educators across a panoply of interprofessional settings are working and learning together on a daily basis. Rather it is argued that educators and learners should approach the concept critically, neither underestimating its complexity nor ignoring the growing evidence base that supports it.

There are a number of key areas that IPL focuses upon: the modification of attitudes; enhancement of communication and collaboration; improvement of services and job satisfaction and the implementation of policy and general change (Barr, 2002). It is argued that IPL is best approached from within an understanding of social learning theory. Learning is thus an on-going process, dynamic and involved with the interaction of individuals; it has a social context. Key aspects of this become opportunities in areas like observation where learners gain an opportunity to witness and observe others.

An understanding of different professional cultures is fundamental to the IPL process; merely sitting in a room with someone from another profession won't work. Similarly, situated learning elements are also seen as fundamental – placing an emphasis on the practice environment. Students should learn in, and from, the community and situations in which they work. IPL should focus on real practice situations and reflect local issues, structures and service delivery. Constructivist learning theory is also important within IPL, based on the notion that learners create their own knowledge and perception of the world, building on their experiences in the construction of new learning indivisible from its social context (Mann et al., 2009). IPL ought to incorporate a relativist (rather than objective) approach; how one views things will depend on where one is stood.

Collaborative learning has obvious merits as a strategy, creating space for learners to learn alongside each other. It should involve a sharing of responsibility and acceptance of a group's actions. A specific illustration of this is problem-based learning where groups of learners are given open-ended problems to be solved in small groups that are facilitated by the educator. The problems tend to be 'real life', authentic scenarios that will drive knowledge and skill acquisition as well as learning and teamworking strategies. A variant, enquiry and action-based learning, is also popular.

Reflection is another key area for educators to consider. Clark (2009) advocates self-assessments (in areas such as personality, learning styles, attitudes to conflict etc.), journaling and written papers looking at stepping back from the professional perspective to reflect upon one's own self. This theme is continued in Axelsson and Axelsson (2009) who consider the issue of IPL and altruism. They suggest working on revealing positive and constructive experiences of accomplishing more together, to enhance altruism at both practitioner and leadership levels. It is better to learn conflict management techniques, such as trading on hierarchies of preferences, than to simply pretend conflict won't exist.

CASE STUDY

Tom is a nurse working in a Community Mental Health Team (CMHT) and is currently on a postgraduate programme of study. He is working towards the completion of his dissertation and has attended research methods teaching at the university. The teaching comes from a range of lecturers from across a broad health and social care background and Tom's classmates are from a similar range of backgrounds, including social work, occupational health nursing and community psychiatric nursing. There are a number of issues surrounding IPL that Tom is reflecting upon:

- Within the CMHT Tom is working with different professional groupings that have significantly different professional cultures and backgrounds. The CMHT is working in an interdisciplinary way to deliver joined up services. Tom is aware of the limits that exist in his team with regard to a 'seamless service'. He feels the team should devote more time to learning about each other's professional backgrounds, culture and understandings. Tom intends to raise this matter at the next staff meeting.
- In the university Tom is learning alongside a range of professionals on a shared learning task looking at good practice in service user involvement in research. He reflects upon which level his IPL is taking place. Tom is finding that there are parallel differences between the medical and social model and between health and social care research.
- The programme delivers learning by drawing upon a range of different scenarios that have meaning to the whole class. Tom reflects upon what arguments there are for having separated (i.e. by professions) elements of the learning given the different traditions in research between health and social care.
- Tom feels that his learning is enhanced by inputs from educators and practitioners with different professional backgrounds. He feels sure that his future practice, learning and research would improve its quality and validity if it incorporated an interprofessional dimension. Tom reflects on whether his colleagues feel the same way.

CONCLUSION

Despite the notable problems facing the construction of a convincing evidence base for IPL, the need for practitioners and educators alike to pursue this agenda is clear. We have identified elements of a growing body of evidence that surrounds IPL and points broadly to learner-centred, situated learning that affords an opportunity to learn with, from and about each other (Barr et al., 2005). The on-going debates about whether IPL evolves from experience ('caught') or can, indeed be learnt ('taught') should not allow educators to ignore the importance of IPL. It is interesting to see that some of the most recent research encourages a closer reflection on our personal rather than professional identity in relation to working with others in order to create better futures for the users of our services. The increasing complexity and specialisation of the work environment ensure that IPL will remain an important issue. If we approach IPL critically, however, and resist seeing it as a panacea, the question will remain as to what balance we draw between learning about our own profession as well as that of others.

See also: experiential and work-based learning; learning styles; partnership working; problem-based learning; reflection; transformative learning

FURTHER READING

Barr, H., Koppel, I., Reeves, S., Hammick, M. and Freeth, D. (2005) *Effective Interprofessional Education: Argument, Assumption and Evidence.* Malden, MA: Blackwell.

REFERENCES

Anning, A. (2005) 'Investigating the impact of working in multi-agency service delivery settings in the UK on early years practitioner's beliefs and practices', *Journal of Childhood Research*, 3: 19–50.

Axelsson, S. and Axelsson, R. (2009) 'From territoriality to altruism in interprofessional collaboration and leadership', *Journal of Interprofessional Care*, 23 (4): 320–30.

Barr, H. (2002) *Interprofessional Education Today, Yesterday and Tomorrow: A Review.* London: Learning and Teaching Support Network.

Barr, H., Koppel, I., Reeves, S., Hammick, M. and Freeth, D. (2005) *Effective Interprofessional Education: Argument, Assumption and Evidence.* Malden, MA: Blackwell.

Care Quality Commission (2009) *Review of the Involvement and Action taken by Health Bodies in Relation to the Case of Baby P.* London: Care Quality Commission.

Clark, P. (2009) 'Reflection on reflection in interprofessional education: implications for theory and practice', *Journal of Interprofessional Care*, 23 (3): 213–23.

Department of Health (2000) *A Health Service of All Talents: Developing an NHS Workforce.* London: HMSO.

Department of Health (2006) *Our Health, Our Care, Our Say.* London: HMSO.

Dutton, A. and Worsley, A. (2009) 'Doves and hawks: practice educators attitudes towards interprofessional learning', *Learning in Health and Social Care*, 8 (3): 145–53.

Easen, P., Atkins, M. and Dyson, P. (2000) 'Interprofessional collaboration and conceptualisations of practice', *Children and Society*, 14: 355–67.

Lord Laming (2003) *The Victoria Climbié Inquiry: Report of an Inquiry by Lord Laming.* London: Department of Health.

Mann, K., Mcfetridge-Durdle, J., Martin-Misener, R., Clovis, J., Rowe, R., Beanlands, H. and Sarria, M. (2009) 'Interprofessional education for students of the health professions: the "seamless care" model', *Journal of Interprofessional Care*, 23 (3): 224–33.

Mattick, K. and Bligh, J. (2006) 'Getting the measure of interprofessional learning', *Medical Education*, 40: 399–400.

Mead, G. (2007) *Walk the Talk: Sustainable Change in post-2000 Interprofessional Learning and Development.* London: Department of Health.

Pollard, K., Miers, M. and Gilchrist, M. (2004) 'Collaborative learning for collaborative working: initial findings from a longitudinal study of Health and Social Care education', *Health and Social Care in the Community*, (12): 346–58.

Salmon, D. and Jones, M. (2001) 'Shaping the interprofessional agenda: a study examining qualified nurse's perceptions of learning with others', *Nurse Education Today*, 21 (1): 18–25.

Walsh, C., Gordon, M., Marshall, M., Wilson, F. and Hunt, T. (2005) 'Interprofessional capability: a developing framework for interprofessional education', *Nurse Education in Practice*, 5 (4): 230–7.

17 leadership and management in academia

Margaret Andrews

DEFINITION

Leadership and management are often viewed as distinct, different and sometimes contradictory concepts. In practice, it is often difficult to distinguish the activities associated with one or the other, and most of us are required to both lead and manage, particularly in relation to organisational change. The extent to which we do either is usually the result of our role requirements, personal perspective and capability. Leadership is about conceptualising a course of action and influencing others to understand and agree on how it can be executed effectively (Yukl, 2002), whereas managing is more to do with the operation of systems, monitoring progress and assessing performance (Bargh et al., 2000). Therefore leaders are usually responsible for creating and sustaining a vision, often for change, and managers are responsible for putting the changes in place and overseeing progress.

The notion that leadership is related to change, particularly in the Higher Education (HE) context, is further explained by Ramsden (1998). Paul Ramsden, currently Chief Executive of the Higher Education Academy in the United Kingdom (UK), indicates that although universities have similar features to other organisations, the fundamental difference lies in the business of education, that is, learning, the product of which is change. The job of academic leaders therefore is to help people change by learning.

Within HE, leadership is often viewed more positively than management, perhaps because leadership is more closely aligned with academic pursuits such as teaching, whereas management has become synonymous with administration, all the less exciting things that academics do to support the educational processes, carrying negative connotations. Often managing is not valued by academics and is seen as getting in the way of the main purpose of education (teaching the subject), negating academic freedom and trivialising what academics do.

There are a number of different styles of leadership and management, based on different assumptions about the nature of individuals and organisations. The style that you will adopt will be based on your beliefs and values, the particular situation, and the nature of the organisation in which you work. Styles of leadership described in the literature include participative, charismatic, situational, transactional and transformative. Particular management styles are more an overall method of leadership used by managers and, in the main, fall into two contrasting approaches: autocratic, which relies on unilateral decision making, and democratic, which supports the involvement of others in decision making. I have put forward an overly simplistic view of management and leadership styles and recommend that you access more informative sources.

To summarise, in contemporary HE, leadership and management are of equal importance, with neither being more valuable than the other. Rather, it is the knowledge of when to apply particular skills and approaches that provides the key to effective leadership and management. For those who are both leaders and managers, many of the differences between leadership and management are blurred because of the tensions between implementing strategic thinking and ensuring that the vision is operationalised in a sustainable way.

KEY POINTS

- Leadership and management are often defined in the literature as being distinct and different, but in practice they overlap.
- Leading is often associated with visioning and leading change and management as more operational (putting changes in place).
- In HE, leadership is seen positively as it is aligned with academic pursuit and managing is seen negatively as it is associated with administration.
- Learning and change are inextricably linked, as change is the product of learning.
- There are a number of styles of leadership and management, which are determined by the nature of the individual, the circumstances and the organisation.

DISCUSSION

This discussion is set against a background of momentous change in HE and everyone who has a leadership or management role will understand just what a challenging and unpredictable time this is. The changes are both within HE itself, for example, the changing nature of the student, and external, such as those associated with funding and culture caused by the global economic recession. The current financial downturn is having an effect on all private and public sector organisations and is likely to do so for the foreseeable future.

Managing and leading in HE have become more complex and demanding, especially in the current climate of diminishing resource, greater emphasis on the student experience and expectations that academics in healthcare should be good teachers, clinicians, administrators and researchers. Alongside this, there is greater pressure from students for more value for money as they increasingly see themselves as 'customers'.

In the UK, the introduction of tuition fees, increasing diversity in the student body and evaluations like the National Student Survey (NSS) have all had an impact on universities and how they position themselves. Increasing differentiation in the HE sector means that for the majority of prospective students there are more choices to be made and with the range of data available, their choices can be better informed, more than ever before.

There is much in the literature about leadership in HE but little relating to management. The leadership literature tends to focus on what leaders do rather than what constitutes effectiveness. Effectiveness may of course depend on who judges it and their perspective and position in the organisation (Bryman, 2009).

Over more recent years there has been a change in the conception of academic leadership. This has paralleled changes in the way that higher education institutions have been managed. Traditionally, universities were not seen as institutions that had to be managed (Bargh et al., 2000). They tended to rely on collegial decision making and often management roles such as head of department were honorary positions and frequently undertaken on a rotational basis. This meant that there was no real motivation for managers to assume the role and many universities offered sabbatical leave to the post holder by way of reward. It was not really until the former polytechnics in the UK joined the university sector in 1992 that this changed; they had a greater tradition of management, which was reflected in their organisational structures.

The challenges

In the UK, non-medical health professional education has been fully within mainstream HE for the past 11 years, with the last of the schools of nursing being integrated in 1998. Across the rest of Europe and more globally the picture is varied, depending on the status of particular professions and the nature of the professional education system within the country. Many leaders/ managers of health professional education have a background in management, with the majority having had clinical leadership roles prior to moving into education (McKimm, 2004). Continuous and rapid changes in health and social care and education mean that many leaders/managers are undertaking new and challenging roles. In 2004 a project examined leadership in medical and healthcare education and highlighted the increasing age profile of health academic leaders (McKimm, 2004). The findings demonstrate that the majority of leaders are clinically qualified, have a higher degree and that there are differences in gender split between medical and non-medical health academic leaders. The former are mostly male whereas the latter are mostly female.

Leading and managing in healthcare education presents its own additional challenges to those generally associated with HE. As well as the generic challenges relating to the interface between teaching, administration and research, there are supplementary ones associated with professional programmes. Examples of these are the different funding and quality assurance arrangements, additional external stakeholder involvement and the need for leaders and managers of health professional education to be both academically and professionally qualified.

CASE STUDY

The following is a real-life case study which focuses on one aspect of leadership, that of choosing and leading a team. Although the context from which this is taken is not wholly located in academic leadership *per se*, it is applicable to a variety of leadership challenges where teams of individuals are involved, for example, leading a module or programme.

In 2008 in an effort to re-focus on the student experience and develop student-focused services that were fit for the future, a university underwent a major change programme and I, together with a group of six others, was responsible for leading this. The change was focused on implementing the recommendations from an external consultancy report following a review of all student-facing services offered. The change team came from a variety of areas in the university and, although known to each other, they had not previously worked together in this way.

One of my first tasks in this leadership role was to bring the individuals together to form the change team. My main concern when forming the team was to ensure that there was a range of expertise and the members were chosen to complement my abilities and characteristics. I had previously undertaken a work profiles questionnaire (Margerison–Mcann Team Management Wheel) to identify what my specific leadership inclinations were. The profile indicated that I worked well at a strategic level and felt comfortable with fairly abstract concepts, therefore it was essential that at least one team member had a propensity for detail and practicality.

This is a significant point: if as a leader you surround yourself with like individuals then it is unlikely that there will be question or challenge, without which, leadership may be ill informed and the project will be less successful.

As the team had not worked together previously and was composed of individuals in a variety of positions in the university, including the President of the Students' Union, it was important to establish the ground rules and clarify roles. Examples of the ground rules by which we operated were:

- commitment – we would wholeheartedly commit to the project and attend all meetings, both formal and informal.
- confidentiality – we would be clear about what was confidential to the team and what was not.
- status – all members including the student representative were full members of the team.
- mutual respect – we had the right to be heard and the right to respectfully challenge each other.

My overall focus throughout the project was to keep hold of the vision for the change (what we set out to do) and to sustain it and influence others to understand and agree their part in the changes (how the change would be executed effectively).

On reflection, leadership of this particular project and with these particular people was a wholly enjoyable experience. An important and memorable moment was getting started – establishing the change team and getting to know each other's strengths, abilities and characteristics. I learnt many lessons including:

- You can't please all the people all of the time.
- Most people can be brought around with the right leadership engagement.
- There are real added benefits of working with colleagues that you don't normally work with, but it is important to be clear about leadership within the team.
- It is important to balance members with different skills and these are advantages in having a student representative as part of the team (they are the real leaders for change in relation to the student experience).
- At times change needs to be driven from the top, but it's nice when the ideas come from the bottom up.

For an account of the project from which this case study emanates please refer to www.heacademy.ac.uk/projects/detail/change_academy_canterbury_2008; for Team Management Profiling refer to www.tmsdi.com.

CONCLUSION

In summary, the nature of management and leadership in healthcare education is challenging and problematic. Although these organisational roles are seen as critical in organisations, there is no real agreement about what managers or leaders should do. As well as the general complexities associated with university leadership and management, for example, aligning tensions between collegial tradition and managerialism, there are others concerning the changing nature of healthcare, increasing demands of a variety of stakeholders such as funding bodies, and the need in some cases to remain clinically active in the absence of agreed clinical academic career structures.

The purpose of this chapter is to make the case that there is a need for competent, flexible, dynamic enthusiastic leaders and managers of HE who can adapt to an uncertain future. Leading and managing in HE is exciting and rewarding, but certainly not for the fainthearted.

See also: academic staff development; management of modules and programmes; partnership working; quality assurance and enhancement; role model

FURTHER READING

Alimo-Metcalfe, B. and Alban-Metcalfe, J. (2005) 'Leadership: time for a new direction?', *Leadership*, 1: 51. Retrieved from http://lea.sagepub.com/cgi/content/abstract/1/1/51

Whitchurch, C. (2008) *Professional Managers in UK Higher Education: Preparing for Complex Futures, Research and Development Series, Final Report*. London: Leadership Foundation for Higher Education.

REFERENCES

Bargh, C., Bocock, J., Scott, P. and Smith, D. (2000) *University Leadership: The Role of the Chief Executive*. Buckingham: The Society for Research into Higher Education.

Bryman, A. (2009) *Effective Leadership in Higher Education*. Research and Development Series, Final Report. London: Leadership Foundation for Higher Education.

McKimm, J. (2004) *Developing Tomorrow's Leaders in Health and Social Care Education: Case Studies in Leadership in Medical and Healthcare Education, Subject Centre Specialist Report 5: FDTL4 Leadership Development Programme*. York: Higher Education Academy.

Ramsden, P. (1998) *Learning to Lead in Higher Education*. London: Routledge.

Yukl, G. (2002) *Leadership in Organisations*, 5th edn. Englewood Cliffs, NJ: Prentice–Hall.

key concepts in
healthcare education

18 learning environments

Annette McIntosh

DEFINITION

The dictionary definition of an environment states that it is to do with the surroundings or conditions in which an individual lives or operates (Oxford English Dictionary, 2009). In an educational context, when the environment, or climate, pertains to the learning and teaching of students, a complex picture is evident, especially in relation to professional education, which includes student experience in practice. Entwistle et al. (2002) considered that the term 'teaching–learning environment' encompassed a broad spectrum of concepts relating to the learning of students involving three levels: social, cultural and political influences; institutional, professional and departmental contexts; and an inner level incorporating the many elements that can directly influence the student experience.

KEY POINTS

- Promotion of effective learning environments requires consideration of multiple concepts, including institutional, professional and programme-based contexts.
- Learning environments perceived as positive by students can facilitate engagement in learning and deep approaches to study.
- Clinical practice is often a key element in healthcare programmes; enhancing positive and supportive learning environments is the joint responsibility of academic staff and practitioners.

DISCUSSION

In order to promote and enhance student learning, there are multiple elements to consider in relation to the environment, both in academic and clinical practice contexts.

Academic learning environments

As noted in Entwistle et al.'s (2002) definition, the learning environment can be seen to be influenced by various levels of factors, from the macro to the micro level. At the macro level, the operation and ethos of a Higher Education

Students and student culture	Course contexts
• Orientations, beliefs, norms and values • Peer groups, morale and identities • Abilities, knowledge and learning skills • Demands and support from outwith the HEI • Learning histories and developmental level	• Course design and organisation • Workload and opportunities for practice • Contact hours and different types of teaching; • Aims and learning outcomes
Teaching and assessing content	**Staff–student relationships**
• Content choice and organization • Teaching methods • Assessment and feedback	• Guidance and support for learning • Affective quality of relationship • Sense of fairness and moral order
Teachers' beliefs, teaching conceptions and reflective practice	

Table 18.1 Entwistle et al.'s 'inner' concepts relating to the learning–teaching environment (adapted from Entwistle et al., 2002: 8)

Institution (HEI) will be affected by the prevailing political, social and cultural contexts, while at the meso level, factors such as institutional, regulatory, professional and disciplinary requirements will influence academic development and delivery. In relation to healthcare, the drivers include professional body requirements, which often provide set conditions that programmes have to meet, both in development and delivery, and which in turn affect the learning environment.

However, as Entwistle et al. (2002) noted, it is the micro level of influences that most directly impacts on students' learning experiences and perceptions; various aspects of the environment can positively or negatively affect the engagement of students in programmes, the adoption of deep approaches to learning and the achievement of high-quality learning outcomes. Research by Lizzio et al. (2002) supported the premise that perceptions of a good environment positively influence both quantitative and qualitative learning outcomes, generic and workplace skills and academic achievement. Entwistle et al. (2002) produced a conceptual framework to guide their research on learning environments, explicating an 'inner' set of concepts that highlight the complexities involved in achieving an effective learning–teaching environment, as shown in Table 18.1, in an adapted format.

As can be seen, each of the concepts has various underpinning elements. Considering the concept of students and their culture in relation to education in healthcare requires recognition that these students often have a different profile from the traditional student entrants to an HEI. The diverse entry gate, especially evident in nursing pre-registration programmes, means that students may come from a wide age range, with differing experiences and level of family commitments. Students will also have to balance the theoretical and practical elements of learning, while coping with the professional socialisation involved in healthcare programmes. At post-registration and postgraduate levels, a further consideration is the creation of a supportive learning environment for part-time students, who are often holding down demanding roles as well as studying for their professional development. All these factors need to be considered in an effort to ensure an appropriate learning environment for healthcare students.

The concepts of programme contexts and teaching and assessing of content include the premise of the necessary constructive alignment of the curriculum, as developed by Biggs (1996). This essentially entails that all elements of the curriculum are compatible and encourage deep learning, with Biggs (1996) describing constructive alignment as the marriage between the constructivist approach to learning and a teaching design featuring alignment of the curriculum. Lizzio et al. (2002) supported the notion that students who perceive a learning environment positively, especially the teaching quality and appropriate assessments, are influenced towards deep approaches to study, while conversely students perceiving a bad learning environment tend towards surface learning approaches.

The relationships between staff and students are important, with the lecturer's own beliefs, teaching stance and reflective practice underpinning many of the elements involved in this concept. In the United Kingdom, the National Union of Students (NUS), in a research report, stated that 'beyond the pedagogic effectiveness, students are particularly positive about lecturers who manage to convey their enthusiasm for a subject, captivating and engaging the students and inspiring them to discuss and research the topic area' (NUS, 2008: 13). Biggs (2003) considered that it is the individual lecturer, as well as the HEI, who creates the climate for learning and noted that this concerns the feelings and perceptions of both students and lecturers, formed through formal and informal interactions. Using McGregor's (1960) theory X (use of control–supervision–punishment) and theory Y (use of guidance–development–reward), Biggs (2003) characterises learning climates as either X or Y: climate X tends to stimulate anxiety and restrict learning, while a climate based on theory Y will encourage deep approaches to learning. It is further noted by Biggs (2003) that whilst learning climates will necessarily contain elements of both X and Y, he not surprisingly advocates a leaning to theory Y, where teachers create a balanced learning climate for optimal learning, taking into account relevant conditions, influences and requirements.

This includes working within the realities, and often constraints, of institutional resources and finances. As Entwistle et al. (2002) observed, while the literature suggests optimum ways of working, these may not be pragmatic or possible due to such pressures of increasing student numbers, depletion of funding and resource constraints, both physical and human. At an operational level, delivery of the curriculum can be shaped by the resources available, the numbers and skill mix of the staff and, in the case of e-learning, the information and communication technological support systems of the HEI. When considering the education of healthcare practitioners, there is also the requirement to provide a safe learning environment for students to practise and develop their skills, including fully equipped skill laboratories.

Ultimately, the quality of the learning environment is a key focus in quality reviews. Within healthcare education, the practice learning environment is under particular scrutiny.

Practice learning environments

Many of the principles associated with ensuring an effective learning environment in the academic context hold true when considering the student experience in practice. Professional learning in practice requires a learning environment conducive to applying theory and developing skills, necessitating support of the student by skilled practitioners and educationalists. As Quinn and Hughes (2007) noted, the experiential learning that takes place in practice can be seen to be more meaningful and relevant than that gained within an HEI setting; creating the right environment is therefore essential.

Support by mentors has been shown to be key in enabling the learning of students, with Lofmark and Wikblad (2001) reporting that factors that obstructed practice learning included staff who lacked interest and did not facilitate reflection on practice.

The learning environment is also influenced by the ethos of a practice area and the attitudes of the qualified staff; the manager has been shown to be particularly influential, including his or her leadership style and personality (Orton, 1981; Papp et al., 2003). Another factor pertaining to the student learning experience in practice is the element of professional socialisation. Studies spanning the past four decades have shown that students assimilate a discipline's norms in an attempt to gain professional identity and that the disparity and conflict between values espoused in the educational context and those in clinical practice can culminate in a 'reality shock' for students (for example, Kramer, 1974; Randle, 2003). This highlights the need for healthcare educationalists and practitioners to work together to foster a supportive learning environment for students; one in which education and learning are valued and facilitated.

CASE STUDY

A multi-professional group of students are undertaking their first module of a postgraduate teaching certificate. The module leader divides the students into small groups with the remit to reflect on and discuss the learning environments within which they work, and then to review a range of literature provided for the purpose.

One group contains Alison, a midwifery practice teacher, Christopher, a lecturer/practitioner in occupational therapy and Lauren, a new social work lecturer. Their initial discussions centre around resource issues, particularly staffing, buildings, rooms, available equipment and information technology systems to support their teaching endeavours. All agree that these are the key elements in ensuring an appropriate learning environment for their students. However, on reviewing the range of literature, the group are surprised to find that the concept is much more complex and multi-factorial than they had realised. Their subsequent discussions focus very much on the student and learning culture, alongside the practical elements of programme organisation and delivery. In particular, they enjoy a debate about their own teaching styles and share their experiences of educators they had found to be very effective in supporting and facilitating their learning. In the plenary feedback session, it is evident that the other groups had had similar initial perceptions and had not realised the broad scope of elements pertaining to learning environments.

CONCLUSION

The concept of the learning environment is a complex one, with many factors contributing to enhancing this aspect of the student experience. A perceived positive learning environment is seen to benefit students' learning and skill development and all those involved in creating and influencing learning environments need to consider all the interacting elements. The requirement for healthcare academics and practitioners is to work collaboratively to support student learning, both in HEI settings and in practice.

See also: curriculum models and design; curriculum planning and development; learning styles; management of modules and programmes; quality assurance and enhancement; student support; teaching strategies; teaching styles

FURTHER READING

Biggs, J.B. (2003) *Teaching for Quality Learning at University: What the Student Does.* Buckingham: SRHE and Open University Press.

REFERENCES

Biggs, J.B. (1996) 'Enhancing teaching through constructive alignment', *Higher Education,* 32: 1–18.
Biggs, J.B. (2003) *Teaching for Quality Learning at University: What the Student Does.* Buckingham: SRHE and Open University Press.
Entwistle, N., McCune, V. and Hounsell, J. (2002) *Approaches to Studying and Perceptions of University Teaching-Learning Environments: Concepts, Measures and Preliminary Findings. Occasional Report 1.* Retrieved from www.etl.tla.ed.ac.uk/docs/ETLreport1.pdf
Kramer, M. (1974) *Reality Shock: Why Nurses Leave Nursing.* London: Mosby.
Lizzio, A., Wilson, K. and Simons, A. (2002) 'University students' perceptions of the learning environment and academic outcomes: implications for theory and practice', *Studies in Higher Education,* 27 (1): 27–52.
Lofmark, A. and Wikblad, K. (2001) 'Facilitating and obstructing factors for development of learning in clinical practice: a student perspective', *Journal of Advanced Nursing,* 34: 43–50.

McGregor, D. (1960) *The Human Side of Enterprise*. New York: McGraw–Hill.

National Union of Students (2008) *Student Experience Report*. Retrieved from the NUS website: www.nus.org.uk/PageFiles/4017/NUS_StudentExperienceReport.pdf

Orton, H. (1981) 'Ward learning climate and student nurse response', *Nursing Times, Occasional Paper No. 17*, 77: 65–8.

Oxford English Dictionary (2009) Retrieved from OED website: www.askoxford.com

Papp, I., Markkanen, M. and von Bonsdorff, M. (2003) 'Clinical environment as a learning environment: student nurses' perceptions concerning clinical learning experiences', *Nurse Education Today*, 23 (4): 262–8.

Quinn, F. and Hughes, S. (2007) *Quinn's Principles and Practice of Nurse Education*, 5th edn. Cheltenham: Nelson Thornes.

Randle, J. (2003) 'Changes in self-esteem during a 3 year pre-registration diploma in higher education (nursing) programme', *Learning in Health and Social Care*, 2 (1): 51–60.

19 learning styles

Moira Hulme and Rob Hulme

key concepts in healthcare education

DEFINITION

Learning styles refer to learners' preferences about the types of learning experience that benefit them most. There is, however, no single definition of the term 'learning styles' and the burgeoning number of theories, models and instruments present a confusing mix to the educator. The terminology of 'learning styles', 'cognitive styles', 'learning strategies' and 'multiple intelligences' is often used imprecisely and interchangeably, to a point where it loses conceptual clarity. The contested nature of learning styles can be crudely summarised in terms of the 'state or trait debate' (Cassidy, 2004). All learning styles theories emphasise *how* students are most likely to learn, rather than *what* they learn, but researchers occupy different positions as to whether learning styles are relatively stable characteristics (a trait or predisposition) or products of our cultural interaction (a situational or environmental state). If learning styles are largely fixed characteristics, educators might enhance learning by 'matching' teaching to individual needs. Conversely, if learning styles are less fixed, learners would benefit from opportunities to develop an extended repertoire of styles.

KEY POINTS

- Learning styles inventories have been used as diagnostic, predictive and pedagogical tools to encourage reflection on learning by students and educators. Discussion of learning styles encourages metacognition ('thinking about thinking').
- The research evidence for learning styles is at best variable. There is little empirical evidence for the *face validity* (that the instrument measures what it claims to measure) and *reliability* (internal consistency and re-test reliability over time) of many models and hence for the practical use of instruments in education settings.
- Critical engagement by practitioners with the evidential base of learning styles is necessary to prevent application of labels that might restrict learner potential and opportunities.

DISCUSSION

Contemporary debates about learning styles are informed by: (a) *political imperatives* to optimise outcomes for learners influenced by ideas about 'human capital' and individual employability; (b) a developing evidence base from *education science*, which draws on cognitive and developmental psychology and neuroscience; and (c) recent trends towards the commodification and marketisation of learning within the current fashion for '*psycho-pedagogy*' (Burton, 2007) traded by educational consultants and training providers 'selling' individual 'remedies' for barriers to learning.

Attention to learning styles received official endorsement from the United Kingdom government as part of its strategy to enhance social justice through *personalised learning* (Leadbetter, 2004). *Learner-centred* pedagogy, curriculum and assessment practices were positioned among a raft of reforms designed to reduce the 'opportunity gap'. Participation in reflection on learning and the development of greater awareness among educators of individual learning styles and the relationship of these to dominant teaching styles were part of a policy ensemble to tackle *equity issues*. It was argued that interventions to promote self knowledge, associated with self efficacy, might improve learner retention and achievement. Moreover, exploration of learning styles might promote greater dialogue between teachers and learners working together as partners in a joint enterprise ('learning conversations'). Responsiveness to learning styles is highlighted in policy documents and inspection reports, confirming its position within the official accounts of 'good practice'. Despite the endorsement and professional application of learning styles, models and measures within education settings, there is considerable controversy about the supporting evidence for these models.

In their review of the literature on learning styles, Coffield et al. (2004) identified 71 theories of learning styles published between 1902 and 2002. Curry

(1983) has organised the diverse array of models and theoretical frameworks on learning styles into three classifications (or 'layers'). The layers in Curry's 'onion model' move from conceptions of learning that are more fluid and open to influence to those that are most stable over time: (1) *instructional preference* or predisposition (for example, some people prefer to work individually, others benefit from collaborative or team-based learning); (2) *information processing* style (the focus here is on learners' habits for storing and retrieving new information); and (3) *cognitive personality* style (fixed inherited characteristics). Broadly speaking, learning styles, theories and models can be located along a continuum stretching from conceptions of individual dispositions to learning as *static* or fixed traits that are stable over time ('hard wired' in the mind) to a view of learning styles as *fluid* and influenced by external factors about where and what is being learned such as the subject culture, curriculum and learning environment.

For educators, the distinction between a fixed learning *style* and flexible learning *strategies* is important. In the design of what is taught and strategies for how it is to be taught, educators can 'design in' learning opportunities that accommodate the different ways individuals learn. Awareness of diverse learning preferences and dispositions reduces the likelihood of a consistent mismatch between how teachers teach and how students learn.

Critical reviews of the literature reveal 'strong' and 'weak' versions of learning styles (Sharp et al., 2008). Strong versions include rigorous attention to the establishment of validity and reliability. Strong research-based versions have developed within the complementary disciplines of cognitive psychology, education and neuroscience, and include the approaches referred to in Table 19.1.

In contrast, 'weak' versions are indicative of the development of 'psychopedagogy' (Burton, 2007) within a broader 'positive psychology' movement. Ecclestone and Hayes (2008) have expressed disquiet over the rise of a 'therapeutic pedagogy', which aims to 'empower' less confident learners to overcome (self-imposed) barriers to the achievement of learning goals without consideration of the wider social context in which learning takes place. The past decade has seen an enormous growth in commercial packages, educational consultants and training providers marketing instruments that will identify learner preferences and dispositions for educators in the public sector. Notable among these is the widespread utilisation of *VAK* (Visual, Auditory and Kinaesthetic/tactile) instruments that identify 'types' of learners, accompanied by an increasingly popular professional discourse on *accelerated learning* (Smith, 1998) and *multiple intelligences* (Gardner, 1999). The concern of the esteem movement to encourage learners to self declare their learning styles might paradoxically result in the restriction of opportunities for some (arguably the least conventionally able students). The attachment of labels that may inhibit learners from venturing beyond their prescribed comfort zone is a limitation of the crude application of VAK terminology in education settings.

Table 19.1 Learning styles and approaches

More fixed learning style	Less fixed learning style
Consistent preference Pre-disposed, physiologically based cognitive style	Learning preferences influenced by a range of factors: environmental, cultural, previous experience, climate for learning, curriculum, impact of tutor
Learning style is a '*biologically and developmentally imposed set of characteristics that make the same teaching method wonderful for some and terrible for others*' (Dunn and Griggs 1988: 3)	A learning style is a '*differential preference for learning, which changes slightly from situation to situation. At the same time, there's some long-term stability in learning style*' (Kolb 2000: 8)
Emphasis on 'matching' teaching and learning styles Dunn and Dunn (1999) *Learning Styles Inventory* assesses learner physiology plus cognitive, affective/emotional and social domains of learning.	Emphasis on 'accommodating' a range of styles through a variety of learning experiences Kolb (1999) *Learning Styles Inventory* identifies four learning styles: converging style (problem solving and decision making), diverging style (imaginative, feeling oriented), assimilating style (more concerned with ideas and concepts than people) and accommodating style (adaptive, intuitive, impatient).
Gregorc's (1982) *Style Delineator* identifies four types of learner: concrete sequential (ordered, practical thorough), abstract sequential (analytical, rational and evaluative), abstract random (sensitive, emotional and spontaneous) and concrete random learners (intuitive, original, independent).	Entwistle (1997) *Approaches and Study Skills Inventory for Students* identifies deep (to understand), strategic (to achieve) and surface (to cope) approaches to learning.
Riding and Rayner (1998) *Cognitive Styles Analysis* organises learning styles according to holist/analyst (cognitive organisation), verbaliser/imager (mental representation) classifications	Honey and Mumford (1992) *Learning Styles Questionnaire* identifies activist (flexible, optimistic), reflector (careful, methodological), theorist (logical, disciplined), and pragmatist (practical, technique oriented) orientations

learning styles

Whilst it may be true that some learners have a dominant learning style, a good education does not limit them to that style or type, but ensures that students have opportunities to strengthen the other learning styles … . In misguided hands, learning styles could become not a means of personalising learning, but a new version of general intelligence that slots learners into preconceived categories and puts unwarranted ceilings on their intellectual development and achievement. (Demos, 2004: 12)

CASE STUDY

Basma has recently returned to college having left school some years previously. She has gathered experience as a part-time care assistant. She is a young mother and is involved in a range of voluntary community activities. Basma is strongly motivated to engage with her programme but lacks confidence, in part due to her previous experiences of formal learning in a school environment. During a well-managed but intensive induction programme, Basma feels overwhelmed by the volume of text-based sources of information. As she embarks on the programme, she struggles with modes of delivery that seem to be about handing down 'academic' knowledge. She is quickly demotivated and struggles to see how her experiences connect with the course. She wants to make a contribution, but feels excluded. As the course progresses, students' learning preferences and teaching strategies are more closely aligned:

- A reliable learning styles inventory is used as a diagnostic assessment tool (e.g. Jackson's Learning Styles Profiler, which identifies initiator, analyst, reasoner, implementer) to support discussion of the different ways in which people learn.
- Students experience a wide range of different teaching and learning strategies that accommodate the varying needs of learners.
- Information is presented in different forms that are accessible to all learners, e.g. visual and verbal (written and spoken).
- Students are supported in expanding the range of strategies they use to support their learning.
- Tutors respond to students' needs and preferences in designing content and blended learning activities.

Basma feels more confident in herself as a learner, develops strategies to enhance her learning and feels able to engage fully with the programme. She feels her experiences are valued and she is able to contribute to her own learning and the learning of others.

CONCLUSION

Learning styles inventories have great appeal for educators seeking to develop more personalised and differentiated approaches to teaching and learning. However, it is important to consider the evidence for the validity and reliability of specific models before making use of these instruments and making changes to programmes based on self-report data. Educators have a professional responsibility to make informed judgements about the warrant of interventions. Educators who adopt an 'inquiry stance' (Cochran-Smith and Lytle, 2009) engage in critical reflection, which encourages the field-testing of instruments and deliberation on their applicability within particular contexts. The uncritical adoption of off-the-shelf to the complex problems of practice does not contribute to professional learning. Care should be taken not to limit the range of learning opportunities or label students according to fixed conceptions of sensory preferences or cognitive style. A commitment to personalisation, the pursuit of strategies to enhance differentiation to engage and motivate all learners is commendable, but should be combined with an equal commitment to evidence-informed professional practice.

See also: research and scholarly activity; teaching strategies

FURTHER READING

Cassidy, S. (2004). 'Learning styles: an overview of theories, models and measures', *Educational Psychology*, 24 (4): 419–44.

Coffield, F., Moseley, D., Hall, E. and Ecclestone, K. (2004) *Learning Styles and Pedagogy on Post 16 Learning: A Systematic and Critical Review*. London: Learning and Skills Development Agency.

REFERENCES

Burton, D. (2007) 'Psycho-pedagogy and personalised learning', *Journal of Education for Teaching*, 33 (1): 5–17.

Cassidy, S. (2004). 'Learning styles: an overview of theories, models and measures', *Educational Psychology*, 24 (4): 419–44.

Coffield, F., Moseley, D., Hall, E. and Ecclestone, K. (2004) *Learning Styles and Pedagogy on Post 16 Learning: A Systematic and Critical Review*. London: Learning and Skills Development Agency.

Cochran-Smith, M. and Lytle, S.L. (eds) (2009) *Inquiry as Stance. Practitioner Research for the Next Generation*. New York: Teacher College Press.

Curry, L. (1983) *An Organisation of Learning Styles Theory and Construct*. ERIC Document No. ED 235185.

Demos (2004) *About Learning: Report of the Learning Working Group*. London: Demos.

Dunn, R. and Griggs, S.A. (1988) *Learning Styles: A Quiet Revolution in American Secondary Schools*. Reston, VA: National Association of Secondary School Principals.

Dunn, R. and Dunn, K. (1999) *The Complete Guide to the Learning Styles Inservice System*. Boston, MA: Allyn and Bacon.

Ecclestone, K. and Hayes, D. (2008) *The Dangerous Rise of Therapeutic Education*. London: Routledge.

Entwistle, N.J. (1997) *The Approaches and Study Skills Inventory for Students (ASSIST)*. Edinburgh: Centre for Research on Learning and Instruction, University of Edinburgh.

Gardner, H. (1999) *Intelligences Reframed: Multiple Intelligences for the 21st Century*. New York: Basic Books.

Gregorc, A.R. (1982) *Style Delineator*. Maynard, MA: Gabriel Systems.

Honey, P. and Mumford, A. (1992) *The Manual of Learning Styles*. Maidenhead: Peter Honey Publications.

Kolb, D.A. (1999) *The Kolb Learning Styles Inventory*. Boston, MA: Hay Group.

Kolb, D.A. (2000) *Facilitator's Guide to Learning*. Boston, MA: Hay/McBer.

Leadbetter, C. (2004) *Personalisation through Participation: A New Script for Public Services*. London: Demos/DfES Innovations Unit.

Riding, R. and Rayner, S. (1998) *Cognitive Styles and Learning Strategies: Understanding Style Differences in Learning and Behaviour*. London: David Fulton.

Sharp, J.G., Bowker, R. and Byrne, J. (2008) 'VAK or VAK-uous? Towards the trivialisation of learning and the death of scholarship', *Research Papers in Education*, 23 (3): 293–314.

Smith, A. (1998) *Accelerated Learning in Practice: Brain-based Methods for Accelerating Motivation and Achievement*. Stafford: Network Educational Press.

learning styles

20 management of modules and programmes

Maureen Wilkins

DEFINITION

There is much debate regarding the distinction between management and leadership and the terms are often used interchangeably. However, the dictionary definitions highlight the distinctions between the two. The Oxford English Dictionary (2009) defines managing as being in charge of, administering and regulating resources, while leading refers to influencing others or events. As Whitehead et al. (2007) note, the activities of a manager encompass operational elements such as planning, budgeting, organising and controlling, but the role is enhanced by the use of effective leadership skills.

The management of programmes or modules will thus include many elements of leadership and individuals in these roles are often called programme or module leaders. Programme leadership involves the overall running of a programme, ensuring that elements are coordinated in order to gain the maximum potential from all personnel involved and the best experience for the students. The role of module leadership involves the organisation and delivery of a module of study, requiring consideration of many aspects, from resource management to student support.

KEY POINTS

- Management of programmes and modules requires a clearly defined structure with capable, motivated and well-organised individuals. Teamwork is essential, if programme management is to be successful and a quality experience for the student.
- There are many key elements to consider in delivering educational provision, including good preparation, fostering an appropriate teaching environment and providing and operating good student support systems.
- Quality assurance and enhancement is important in the development and delivery of healthcare programmes at all levels and there are responsibilities in this respect for the institution, programme and module leaders and all academic and support staff.

106

DISCUSSION

Managing modules and programmes effectively requires that the Higher Education Institution (HEI) has the appropriate infrastructure in place to support the process, including well-defined operational procedures and protocols, learning and physical resources and information technologies.

Many studies have demonstrated that the management of programmes and modules plays an important part in the student experience. For example, Yorke and Longden (2008) reported that organisation of provision was highly influential for the students' non-completion in their study. Aspects such as lack of organisation, cancelled sessions and delays in provision of support were shown have negative influences and Yorke and Longden (2008) stated that students need to have clear expectations of a programme, including its limitations, and to know that they themselves will be treated with respect and consideration.

Programme management

In programme management, being involved in the development of the curriculum can be a great advantage in understanding the philosophy and framework of the programme, alongside building relationships with the staff involved, including students, service colleagues and service users and carers. Management of the programme involves many elements from the recruitment and admission of students through to evaluating the effectiveness of the delivery of the provision.

The programme leader is responsible for further developing the curriculum of new programmes post-validation. Biggs (2003) discussed the importance of constructive alignment, based on the twin principles of constructivism in learning and alignment in teaching. For a programme to be successfully managed, all components need to be aligned with each other, horizontally and vertically. Teaching and assessment methods and learning activities have to be developed to ensure that all elements work together to support appropriate learning. In this endeavour, Quinn and Hughes (2007) note the usefulness of schedules of work, or module plans, to guide programme and module delivery as useful tools. These can help ensure that all key components have been covered, and that unnecessary repetition does not occur. In addition, and on an on-going basis, management of the curriculum requires that emerging drivers and initiatives are mapped into and across the programmes to ensure that the provision remains up to date and relevant.

Managing delivery in relation to resources, budget and administration is also key in assuring and enhancing the quality of a programme. This includes ensuring that lecturing staff have the appropriate knowledge and skills to deliver the programme and that acceptable student:staff ratios are maintained, alongside fair staff workloads. Consideration must be given to new lecturers who may require development and mentoring, and the use of visiting specialists and involvement of service users and carers has to be coordinated and managed within budgetary restrictions.

In the management of the learning environment, relationships between staff and students are important. Students should be taught in an environment where learning can be facilitated and encouraged within a non-threatening atmosphere (Lizzio et al., 2002). There is much the programme leader can do to promote an ethos that encourages student engagement and support, including ensuring clear communication of all elements of the provision and developing and allocating Personal Academic Tutors (PATs) for the pastoral support of students (Welsh and Swann, 2002). The programme leader has the overview of a student cohort's progress and educational experiences throughout their programme and is therefore in a position to manage this to the benefit of all involved, notwithstanding the challenges often present in terms of budget and resource constraints.

In many healthcare programmes, students are required to experience learning in practice. Access to quality placements is therefore essential and appropriate clinical experiences should be organised with reference to the curriculum and stage of learning in order to ensure the student has the knowledge and skills to gain the optimum learning experience within the practice area (Glen and Parker, 2003). This involves partnership working with placement providers and requires a cooperative and proactive approach. The HEI also has to have the appropriate administrative systems in place to manage the placement allocation and quality assurance processes.

Management of programmes involves continuous quality monitoring and enhancement in response to external and internal benchmarks and feedback and evaluations. Practical elements for a programme leader in this respect can include forming a programme management team, chairing assessment boards, organising student–staff liaison forums and programme committees, with service user and student representation. It will also entail evidencing the quality of the programme through written reports and participation in internal and external reviews.

Ultimately, the programme leader has a pivotal role in the management of the overall learning experiences for students; module leaders also have important roles to play in this respect.

Module management

Many responsibilities of the module leader are similar to those of a programme leader, but on a smaller scale. In preparing the module for delivery, adherence to the notion of constructive alignment (Biggs, 2003) requires that assessments align with the curriculum content and methods of delivery and that the module handbook and information clearly communicates this to students. Module leaders have the responsibility for producing lesson plans for each session, ensuring that all module content is delivered through formal or informal learning processes and that the content is relevant, current and appropriate to the level of learning. Module leaders need to organise support for students, particularly in relation to the assessment processes, and involvement in quality processes is required; these range from operating the marking and feedback processes to producing reflective module reports that include analysis of trends of student performance and evaluations.

On a practical level, the coordination of the timetable (including room booking) is important, with a logical progression of subjects, study periods and a mix of learning strategies, aligned and complementary to any concurrent modules. The production of material to support the module delivery, such as handbooks, guided study and online materials, requires forward planning and administrative support. Incorporating relevant clinicians, practice educators, specialist practitioners and service users and carers to participate in the delivery of the module can enhance the student learning experience and help to align curriculum content, ensuring relevance to practice (Quinn and Hughes, 2007). Overall, the role can be an excellent opportunity for individual development of new lecturers, though imperative in this is mentoring and peer support.

Common to both module and programme management is the importance of evaluating the provision.

Evaluations

Evaluation is a systematic collection and analysis of information about how successful a programme, module, study day etc. has been as part of the students' learning experience (Neary, 2001). Hounsell (2009) notes that there are three principal sources of feedback: from students; from teaching colleagues and peers; and from self reflection by an individual or team. The use of at least two of these sources is necessary for evaluation to be robust, systematic and meaningful and the timing of evaluation feedback is important. As Hounsell (2009) states, leaving evaluation until the end of a programme is a questionable, though widespread, practice. For module and programme managers to be reflexive to feedback, the process of continuous evaluation is more valuable. The response to evaluations is equally important and students need to know that the information gained will inform future delivery and development, where possible and relevant.

CASE STUDY

Gail has been employed as a lecturer for the past four months following several years of teaching experience as a practice educator. She has just been appointed as leader for a mentorship module, delivered on the main campus. This module is also delivered in four other venues. She reads all the documentation before contacting the other module leaders, suggesting a meeting to ensure her understanding of the module. At the meeting, it is evident that all the necessary documentation, shared lesson plans and assignments have been agreed and that all Gail will be required to manage is classroom booking and the delivery of the module. A member of the module team agrees to act as a mentor to Gail, ensuring she is supported in this new role.

Tony is an experienced senior lecturer; he has had the role of programme leader for the past year and as part of this has to produce the programme annual monitoring review (AMR). He has received all the module reports, including student evaluations and the comments from the external examiners. As he is completing the AMR for the first time, he seeks advice and guidance from the HEI's academic quality support department, to ensure this important document is completed in the appropriate manner. He finds the process challenging, but ultimately it allows him the opportunity to reflect on the strengths and weaknesses of the programme which he takes forward to address with his programme management team.

CONCLUSION

There are many responsibilities and underpinning elements that must be considered by programme and module leaders, with both roles continually interacting to enhance student knowledge, support, development and achievement. The roles involve ensuring that curriculum alignment is managed and the standards required by the HEI are achieved, delivering a quality programme that meets the needs of all students and stakeholders.

See also: curriculum models and design; curriculum planning and development; leadership and management in academia; quality assurance and enhancement; teaching strategies

FURTHER READING

Fry, H., Ketteridge, S. and Marshall, S. (2009) *A Handbook for Teaching and Learning in Higher Education*, 3rd edn. Londen: Routledge.
Neary, M. (2001) *Teaching, Assessing and Evaluation for Clinical Competence. A Practical Guide for Practitioners and Teachers.* Cheltenham: Nelson Thornes.

REFERENCES

Biggs, J.B. (2003) *Teaching for Quality Learning at University: What the Student Does.* Buckingham: SRHE and Open University Press.
Glen, S. and Parker, P. (2003) *Supporting Learning in Practice: A Guide for Practitioners.* Basingstoke: Palgrave Macmillan.
Hounsell, D. (2009) 'Evaluating courses and teaching', in H. Fry, S. Ketteridge and S. Marshall, *A Handbook for Teaching and Learning in Higher Education*, 3rd edn. London: Routledge. pp, 198–213.
Lizzio, A., Wilson, K. and Simons, R. (2002) 'University students' perceptions of the learning environment and academic outcomes: implications for theory and practice', *Studies in Higher Education*, 27 (1): 27–52.
Neary, M. (2001) *Teaching, Assessing and Evaluation for Clinical Competence. A Practical Guide for Practitioners and Teachers.* Cheltenham: Nelson Thornes.
Oxford English Dictionary (2009) Retrieved from OED website: www.askoxford.com
Quinn, F.M. and Hughes, S.J (2007) *Principles and Practices of Nurse Education*, 5th edn. Cheltenham: Nelson Thornes.

key concepts in healthcare education

Welsh, I. and Swann, C. (2002) *Partners in Learning: A Guide to Support and Assessment in Nurse Education*. Abingdon: Radcliffe Medical Press.

Whitehead, D.K, Weiss, S.A. and Tappen, R.M. (2007) *Essentials of Nursing Leadership and Management*, 4th edn. Philadelphia, PA: F.A. Davis.

Yorke, M. and Longden, B. (2008) *The First-Year Experience of Higher Education in the UK: Final Report*. York: Higher Education Academy.

21 mastery

Peter Bradshaw

DEFINITION

The Mastery inherent in the achievement of Masters Degree has certain characteristics that define its purpose. It is firstly a next step for those who have normally achieved a good honours degree. Within its process the candidate will be expected to achieve a specialised knowledge of a specific intellectual domain and, in particular, the Mastery of the conceptual basis of the topic under consideration. Having the ability to think conceptually and to manipulate and apply theoretical propositions is, therefore, a pre-requisite to the achievement of Mastery.

Secondly, in professional practice disciplines and fields of study, candidates are required to create synergies between the intellectual domain and their own personal practice. This occurs in two-way fashion. Taught material is used to shed light on practice but also practical experience is used to enhance learning by creating analogies that assist the interpretation of knowledge. By these processes Mastery is defined by the ability to analyse and synthesise ideas and to develop criticality. The Masters student thus becomes a natural problem solver who treats knowledge and practice as problematic in becoming a more autonomous learner.

KEY POINTS

- The key components of Mastery are truth, knowledge, objectivity and rationality, comprising Mastery of thought.
- The spirit of enquiry is fundamental in understanding Mastery.
- Masters study enhances students' practical experience.

DISCUSSION

The rise of the Masters degree

The development of Masters level education has increased exponentially as part of the rise of credentialism internationally. The requirements of the employment market and of an individual's social status as the 20th century progressed began to demand a more intellectually rigorous range of qualifications (Collins, 1979). Similarly, as a means to a professional qualification, more occupational groups increased their requirements. The female perceived semi-professions of nursing, teaching and social work are examples of this where what had been regarded as practically oriented crafts were reinterpreted by their own members as needing a more educated membership with recognisable academic awards. After an initial requirement for a diploma, degree status usually followed and inevitably there was then a call for Masters level opportunity (Eraut, 1994). Governments, employers and professional bodies embodied this requirement within their policies and universities not only met the initial demand but were to fuel it by marketing an ever-extending range of options.

An additional trend has also been influential in the past 50 years and this concerns continuous professional development (CPD) and lifelong learning. The requirement for the acknowledgement of these has now become a widely accepted occupational norm. Thus for reasons of personal and professional prestige as well as in the interests of career progression, the Masters degree is regarded as an essential. Not only has the focus of the Masters degree changed but also its target audience, who are often experienced professionals with established careers aiming to improve their skills and knowledge (Drennan and Hyde, 2008).

This has meant that the nature of the Masters experience is also evolving and what was formally an academic exercise is now vocationally oriented and increasingly connected to the workplace (Fischer, 2000). So Mastery in the workplace is a critical component in employability and is a function of learning and of bilateral knowledge transference between higher education and the workplace (Aamodt and Havnes, 2008). This means that Mastery embodies what historically were regarded as both education and training. The distinction between them is semantic but while Mastery is concerned with the quality of intellectual and cognitive decisions that are made, preparation for it should be equally cognisant of the psychomotor domain within it by enabling students to 'do' practical things better.

The experience of many occupations is that the newly qualified recruit is fit to be awarded a professional qualification and has fulfilled a level of competence to be able to perform at an acceptable level. Yet the demands of the job may be such that fitness for purpose over a career requires continuous updating and the ability to become an autonomous learner, which is the hallmark of Mastery

The key components for Mastery

The quest for truth, knowledge and objectivity

Seeking truth through deriving cognitive meaning from seemingly objective facts is vital to the achievement of Mastery. The parameters that influence this are evidence, reference, meaning and intention, all of which become central to the student's intellectual journey and experience and which shape ideas, a consequence of which is that the student begins to see things differently (Quine, 1990).

Integral to the quest for truth is objective knowledge (Kuhn, 1996). Objectivity is an elusive concept that is much debated philosophically, but in general terms its contribution to Mastery is that it arises from systematically discovered facts. It is thus discovered by the student rather than being created on the basis of intuition. By adding knowledge to objectivity, there are grounds for a justified truth. The skills required to acquire objective knowledge therefore enhance Mastery by fostering perceptiveness, communication, powers of reasoning and the enhancement of overall understandings of the subject under scrutiny.

Rationality

Rationality refers to the cognitive ability to analyse particular proposals. In practice, rational argument occurs within a logical framework comprising set propositions or premises. Within the process, individuals use strategies that envisage and surmise the problem or issue, balance the evidence and evaluate it and then specify conclusions that form the logical consequences of the process of rational argument (Hanson, 1997). The logical consequence is the association that is drawn between the premises and the conclusion of a valid argument. It can be seen therefore that logical validity is a necessary condition for rationality.

In achieving Mastery students are exposed to a deliberate range of eventualities that nurture and enhance rational thought. There is the interaction with others such as tutors and peers. Students will be required to demonstrate rational argument in their written work as well as through the ability to sustain verbal debate with their fellow students and be evaluated by them. This requires the capacity to interact with and encounter views with which they do not necessarily concur, but have to tolerate. This also demands taking responsibility for any claims they themselves make, all of which exposes the ethical dimension of scholarly debate.

Going a stage further on the road to, and a prerequisite for, Mastery and for rational thought is that students should increasingly examine and question their own beliefs, resulting in the exposure of their own ideas to intellectual self-scrutiny. Schon, a founding initiator of the concept of reflection, suggests the development of the aptitude to reflect *in* action (instantaneous reflection) and *on* action (retrospective reflection) has become an important feature of professional Mastery, notably for its contribution to the need for CPD (Schon, 1983).

The spirit of enquiry

All of the preceding observations lay the foundations for the student who, in developing Mastery, will be acutely attuned to research and enquiry as a component of life. All notions of enquiry test the extent of common sense by examining its limits and extending its explanatory power through empiricism of one form or another. Mastery occurs when the student is familiar with the nuances of a range of techniques. Research training for the attainment of Mastery usually has two principal foci.

Firstly, positivist research, which has its origins in the physical sciences, sets out with very clear goals, precise quantitative measuring devices and large representative samples of respondents. This kind of research employs designs such as randomised controlled trials, experiments and surveys. Structured tools are used that measure statistical differences between variables. The principal objectives of work in this genre are to achieve *reliability*, meaning replication is possible, and *validity*, which indicates the research has measured the phenomena it intended to measure (Byrne, 2002). This type of research intends to establish causal relationships through a dispassionate, unprejudiced investigation in which the researcher is value-free and the purpose is usually to generalise the results to like populations elsewhere (Peat et al., 2002). Although quantitative techniques have broad adherents they have been criticised from within the scientific community, the most notable critic being Popper, who argued that even this most reputable of techniques is capable of false assumptions and could be subject to refutation (Popper, 1975).

A second category of investigation, namely interpretative, also needs to be grasped. These approaches use qualitative techniques and have their origins in the social and behavioural sciences in which their exponents contend that the social world cannot be properly understood by numerical phenomena and that to try to do so is reductionist. The emphasis here is on social reality and on capturing the intricacies of human experience (Parahoo, 2006). This research is interested in values, attitudes, beliefs and human interactions and in examining these, accepts that the researcher's subjective influence on the research process is a given. Unlike the previous paradigm, in this tradition the researcher has less certainty about what will be discovered and hence the research design is less rigid at the outset (Gomm, 2004). Smaller samples of respondents are used, typically for fieldwork using questionnaires, interviews and inventories to capture the meanings in a natural setting; the researcher is the primary medium in data collection and analysis and becomes immersed personally in these activities (Merriam, 1988). Findings that are rich in meaning are accrued and these are reported predominantly in words and the researcher is reliant on the meanings readers draw from the work for any generalisations that come from it (Gomm, 2004). The twin concepts of reliability and validity are inapplicable to qualitative research; rather its veracity is established by the demonstration of the following (Lincoln and Guber, 1985):

Credibility – its plausibility
Transferability – its applicability elsewhere
Dependability – its accurate capture of the context in which the researcher did the study
Confirmability – whether its results are likely to be confirmed by others

History has seen positivist research as emblematic of truthfulness and as the true generator of the laws of theoretical prediction (Peat et al., 2002). A more contemporary view would hold, however, that all well-executed analytical investigation, be it positivist or interpretivist, is a legitimate scholarly endeavour (Bowling and Shah, 2005).

Mastery will inevitably lead to an allegiance and a thorough comprehension of a particular research tradition. Indeed, a critical criterion in assessing Masters-worthiness is to ask if the students have satisfactorily demonstrated undergoing an adequately rigorous programme of research training.

CASE STUDY

The empirical evidence establishes that, for Masters level study, the proof of the pudding is in the eating. A range of evidence is available that has evaluated the student experience. The principal findings in a British study were that Masters study enhances the legitimacy of the profession of nursing, it enhances clinical credibility and authority and the Masters graduate is seen to exercise leadership in a way that enhances the status of the profession (Gerrish et al., 2003).

Positive benefits were also reported in Canadian work. Successful graduates believed themselves to have entered a new reality, have more self confidence, a broader grasp of policy issues and greater professional pride (Cragg and Andrusyszyn, 2004).

In perhaps the most rigorous study, students were surveyed about their professional destinations after graduation (Drennan, 2008). The vast majority had been promoted, but were still in practice, thus reversing a trend seen in Ireland and the UK in the 1990s in which the majority of graduates followed career pathways in nurse education. A minority indicated a wish to study further and those that did were either pursuing a PhD or intended to do so. The overwhelming outcome was the confidence the experience had given them.

CONCLUSION

The evidence relating to Mastery is indeed heartening to the student and prospective student and makes the achievement of Mastery to be a highly worthwhile professional and personal goal.

See also: *academic staff development; research and scholarly activity; supervising Masters and PhD students*

FURTHER READING

Denby, N., Butroyd, R., Swift, H.D., Price, J. and Glazzard, J. (2008) *Masters Level Study in Education: A Guide to Success for PGCE Students*. Milton Keynes: Open University Press.

REFERENCES

Aamodt, P.O. and Havnes, A. (2008) 'Factors affecting professional job mastery: quality of study or work experience?',*Quality in Higher Education*, 14: 233–48.

Bowling, A.and Shah, E. (2005) *Handbook for Health Research Methods: Investigation, Measurement and Analysis*. Buckingham: Open University Press.

Byrne, D. (2002) *Interpreting Quantitative Data*. London: Sage.

Collins, R. (1979) *The Credential Society: An Historical Sociology of Education and Stratification*. London: Academic Press.

Cragg, C.E. and Andrusyszyn, M.A. (2004) 'Outcomes of Masters education in nursing'. *International Journal of Nursing Scholarship*, 1 (1): 1–18.

Drennan, J. (2008) 'Professional and academic destination of masters in nursing graduates: a national survey', *Nurse Education Today*, 28 (16): 751–9.

Drennan, J. and Hyde, A. (2008) 'Social selection and professional regulation for Master's degrees for nurses', *Journal of Advanced Nursing*, 63 (5): 486–93.

Eraut, M. (1994) *Developing Professional Knowledge and Competence*. London: Falmer Press.

Fischer, G. (2000). 'Lifelong learning – more than training', *Journal of Interactive Learning Research*, 11 (3): 265–94.

Gerrish, K., McManus, M. and Ashworth, P. (2003) 'Creating what sort of a professional? Masters level education as professionalising strategy', *Nursing Inquiry*, 10 (2): 103–12.

Gomm, R. (2004) *Social Research Methodology: A Critical Introduction*. Basingstoke: Palgrave Macmillan.

Hanson, W.H. (1997) 'The concept of logical consequence', *The Philosophical Review*, 106: 365–409.

Kuhn, T.S. (1996) *The Structure of Scientific Revolutions*. Chicago: University of Chicago Press.

Lincoln, Y. and Guber, E. (1985) *Naturalistic Inquiry*. Beverley Hills, CA: Sage.

Merriam, S.B. (1988). *Case Study Research in Education: A Qualitative Approach*. San Francisco: Jossey–Bass.

Parahoo, K. (2006) *Nursing Research: Principles, Processes and Issues*. Basingstoke: Palgrave Macmillan.

Peat, J., Mellis, C., Williams, K. and Xuan, W.(2002) *Health Science Research: A Handbook of Quantitative Methods*. London: Sage.

Popper, K.R. (1975) 'The rationality of scientific revolutions', in R. Harré (ed.), *Problems of Scientific Revolution: Scientific Progress and Obstacles to Progress in the Sciences*. Oxford: Clarendon Press.

Quine, W.V. (1990) *Pursuit of Truth*. Cambridge, MA: Harvard University Press.

Schon, D.A. (1983) *The Reflective Practitioner: How Professionals Think in Action*. London: Temple Smith.

key concepts in
healthcare education

Morag Gray

DEFINITION

A mentor is someone who:

> gives wise advice … . In practice, mentors provide a spectrum of learning and supportive behaviours, from challenging and being a critical friend to being a role model, from helping to build networks and develop resourcefulness to simply being there to listen, from helping people work out what they want to achieve, and why, to planning how they will bring change about. (Clutterbuck, 2004: 3)

KEY POINTS

- Effective mentors and mentees demonstrate a range of interpersonal and professional characteristics.
- The relationship between mentor and mentee is of prime importance.
- Mentorship raises several challenges in practice.

DISCUSSION

Historical context

The term mentor originates from Homer's Odyssey, in which Odysseus appointed his old and trusted friend Mentor to be a guide, teacher and adviser to his son while he was away at war. Since the mid 1970s there has been a growing body of literature on mentorship with a particular surge of publications in the past 15–20 years. In the business world in the United States of America, interviews with 40 men identified the most important developmental relationship in their early careers as the one with their mentors (Levinson, 1978). Literature from a wide range of disciplines refers to the use of mentoring to assist career development, to facilitate and support both high and low achievers to reach their potential, and to progress into their chosen careers.

Characteristics of effective mentorship

Mentors are said to promote professional and personal development, which improves and maintains the quality of work the mentee is engaged in and sustains their skill and knowledge base. Clutterbuck (2004: 53) provides a useful mnemonic of the role:

Manages the relationship
Encourages
Nurtures
Teaches
Offers mutual support
Responds to the mentee's needs

Effective mentor relationships are characterised by both parties having a desire to make the relationship work and making a commitment by investing time, emotional energy, honesty, trust, integrity and focusing on the common goals of personal and professional growth and development. Effective mentors exhibit a variety of interpersonal and professional characteristics, as shown in Table 22.1.

Equally, there are characteristics of individuals who make effective mentees (see Table 22.2).

Table 22.1 Interpersonal and professional characteristics of effective mentors

Interpersonal	Professional
• Professionally nurturing independence whilst providing guidance	• Professionally focused helping students develop their professional identity
• A good listener	• Knowledgeable and competent
• Trustworthy	• Upholds standards of excellence in their field
• Interested; empathetic	• Exemplary role model
• Fair, balances praise and criticism	• Creative
• Available and committed to mentoring	• Motivated
• Flexible	• Honest
• Generous	• Organised
• Friendly – accepts mentee as part of team	• Decisive
• Communicative – shares knowledge and expertise	• Hard-working
• Supportive	• Attentive
• Patient	• Responsive
• Considerate	• Non-judgemental and ethical
	• Ability and willingness to facilitate learning in others as a catalyst for growth
	• Ability to facilitate discussion and reflection on practice
	• Ability and willingness to provide honest constructive feedback

Sources: Gray and Smith, 1999, 2000; Haines, 2003; Morton-Cooper and Palmer, 2000; Rose et al., 2005

Table 22.2 Interpersonal and professional characteristics of effective mentees

Interpersonal	Professional
• Eager to grow and learn • Good listener • Committed • Asks for feedback • Enthusiastic • Curious • Ambitious • Communicative • Appreciative • Patient • Respectful of time and effort put in by mentor • Recognises mentor's possible time constraints and conflicting priorities	• Motivated – acts on information provided by mentor • Focused • Goal-driven – invests time and energy • Honest • Open to feedback and perspectives • Willing to undertake new challenges • Hard-working • Responsible • Ready, over time, to become independent

Sources: Gray and Smith, 1999, 2000; Haines, 2003; Morton-Cooper and Palmer, 2000; Rose et al., 2005

Relationships

The emphasis of any mentoring relationship should be a drive to make it successful, ensuring that the benefits outweigh any negative effects. There are a number of challenges associated with ensuring that the mentor–student relationship is a healthy and productive one. The negative side has been under-studied and it is only recently that the dysfunctional relationships that can occur have been acknowledged. Problems include possessiveness, overprotection, oppressive control, exploitation of the student; creating over-dependence and unrealistic expectations (Eby and Allen, 2002; Gray and Smith, 1999, 2000). Mentors should engage in self evaluation, as well as receive feedback on their role from students and their peers, in order to remain alert to these potential challenges.

Parsole and Wray (2000) propose seven golden rules for mentors:

1 Success comes from doing simple things consistently – don't over complicate.
2 Make sure you meet – timetable this into your work.
3 Keep it brief – don't waste time and keep focused.
4 Stick to the basic process.
5 Develop the 'ask' and not 'tell' habit.
6 Remember it's all about learning.
7 Expect to gain yourself.

The relationship should be a negotiated one, and Donaldson and Carter (2005) advise that setting ground rules between mentor and student is important to manage each person's expectation of the other.

Table 22.3   Characteristics of a positive practice learning environment

- Placement is well organised
- Staff share the same philosophy of care
- Students feel that the standard of care is high
- Staff work as an effective and cohesive team
- Staff are approachable, knowledgeable, enthusiastic and supportive
- Staff engender confidence in the student
- The atmosphere is relaxed and student-friendly
- Staff have realistic ideas regarding what students can do at certain stages of their programme
- Students' learning is seen by staff as very important and facilitated in a number of ways – clear explanations, willingness to answer questions even when busy and providing good role models for the students
- Teaching programmes and learning materials are available
- The staff's teaching skills are appreciated and support for students learning new skills
- A key feature is that staff are committed to teaching; they trust and allow students to participate in care independently

Developing the learning environment

A key role within mentoring is creating and managing a good learning environment. This is not a static concept but a dynamic outcome of the interrelationships of a variety of elements that are ever-changing (see Table 22.3).

There is evidence that students experiencing a poor learning environment exhibit signs of vulnerability, anxiety, limited learning and withdrawal from their course (Beskine, 2009; Moscaritolo, 2009). Supporting students in practice is the essence of mentoring. Practice-based learning is about assisting students to apply their theoretical knowledge within the practice setting and to acquire the skills and knowledge required to function as healthcare professionals.

Assessment

Mentors are the gatekeepers of professional standards and they need to challenge students in a supportive way, avoiding the halo effect (the assessor favouring or disfavouring the person being assessed) and failure to fail. To avoid failing to fail (Duffy, 2003) mentors need to be confident in their assessment and feedback skills, and they require support from link lecturers and practice education facilitators (Fulton et al., 2007).

Challenges

It is not surprising that with the scope and complexity of the mentorship role, there are a number of challenges. With increasing student numbers, finding sufficient placements can be difficult and this is further compounded by sickness, holidays and 12-hour shift patterns. However, the latter can be ameliorated through team or co-mentoring. As well as having to achieve an approved mentor preparation programme there is the additional challenge of being released from duty in order to attend annual updates. It is imperative that mentors keep up to date, both in terms of their knowledge, skills and competence and knowledge of their students' programme of study. Time is another challenge in the process of mentoring, particularly when providing patient care and meeting other commitments (Fulton et al., 2007; Gray, 1997). To address this issue, Beskine (2009) asserts that protected non-clinical time should be factored into the mentor's workload.

CASE STUDY

Maggie has two years' experience of mentoring students and she recently encountered her first 'failing' student. Maggie takes her mentor role seriously and what follows are her reflections on how she will deal with the situation.

It's coming up to Gwyneth's mid-placement formative assessment and I need to address her lack of professionalism in the way she communicates with patients and other members of the team. I probably should have said something before now but I can't let it go beyond her mid-placement assessment as then it will be too late to help her. If I don't say anything now, I will condone Gwyneth's bad practice – gosh, what a responsibility this is!

I have planned what I am going to say to Gwyneth but I will get her to self-assess first to see if she has any insight into the problem. That way, it will be easier for us to work together on a realistic action plan to improve her communication skills and meet her placement learning outcomes. If she isn't aware of her communication difficulties, I will talk her through two or three recent, clear examples of occasions when her communications skills were either lacking or inappropriate to help her see where the difficulties lie and how we can work together to help improve her performance. Once we have discussed that, I will get her to draft an action plan (she needs to take ownership of the problem and how to rectify it) and arrange regular meetings so we are both aware of progress being made. I will also need to tell Gwyneth that if she doesn't improve over the next two weeks, I will need to inform the Practice Education Facilitator so that additional support can be put in place as appropriate.

If this kind of situation happens again I really must deal with it straight away rather than waiting and hoping that it will sort itself out! That way it will be much easier to manage, and be fairer on students as they will have longer to rectify their limitations.

CONCLUSION

Perhaps the best way to conclude is to refer to the following ancient Chinese proverb:

If you want 1 year of prosperity, grow grain.
If you want 10 years of prosperity, grow trees.
If you want 100 years of prosperity, grow people.

Mentorship is all about nurturing people to grow – both the mentor and the mentee.

See also: assessment; clinical competence; dealing with failing and problem students; experiential and work-based learning; learning environments; partnership working; practice teaching; teaching styles

FURTHER READING

Connor, M. and Pokora, J. (2007) *Coaching and Mentoring at Work: Developing Effective Practice*. London: Open University Press and McGraw–Hill.

Gopee, N. (2008) *Mentoring and Supervision in Healthcare*. London: Sage.

REFERENCES

Beskine, D. (2009) 'Mentoring students: establishing effective working relationships', *Nursing Standard*, 23 (30): 35–40.

Clutterbuck, D. (2004) *Everyone Needs a Mentor*. London: Chartered Institute of Personnel and Development.

Donaldson, J. and Carter, D. (2005) 'The value of role modelling: perceptions of undergraduate and diploma nursing (adult) students', *Nurse Education in Practice*, 5 (6): 353–9.

Duffy, K. (2003) *Failing Students: A Qualitative Study of Factors that Influence the Decisions Regarding Assessment of Students' Competence in Practice*. Retrieved from NMC website: www.nmc-uk.org/aDisplayDocument.aspx?documentID=1330

Eby, L.T. and Allen, T.D. (2002) 'Further investigation of protégés' negative mentoring experiences: patterns and outcomes', *Group and Organisational Management*, 27 (4): 456–79.

Fulton, J., Bohler, A., Hansen, G.S., Kauffeldt, A., Welander, E., Santos, M.R., Thorarinsdottir, K. and Ziarko, E. (2007) 'Mentorship: an international perspective', *Nurse Education in Practice*, 7 (6): 399–406.

Gray, M.A. (1997) The Professional Socialisation of Project 2000 Student Nurses: A longitudinal qualitative investigation into the effect(s) of supernumerary status and mentorship on student nurses. Unpublished PhD thesis, Department of Nursing and Midwifery, Faculty of Medicine, University of Glasgow.

Gray, M.A. and Smith, L.N. (1999) 'The professional socialisation of diploma of higher education in nursing students (Project 2000): a longitudinal qualitative study', *Journal of Advanced Nursing*, 29 (3): 639–47.

Gray, M.A. and Smith, L.N. (2000) 'The qualities of an effective mentor from the student nurse's perspective: findings from a longitudinal qualitative study', *Journal of Advanced Nursing*, 32 (6): 1542–9.

Haines, S.T. (2003) 'The mentor–protégé relationship', *American Journal of Pharmaceutical Education*, 67 (3): 1–7.

Levinson, D. (1978) *The Seasons of a Man's Life*. New York: Ballantine.

Morton-Cooper, A. and Palmer, A. (2000) *Mentoring, Preceptorship and Clinical Supervision: A Guide to Professional Roles in Clinical Practice*. Oxford: Blackwell Science.

Moscaritolo, L.M. (2009) 'Interventional strategies to decrease nursing student anxiety in the clinical learning environment', *Journal of Nursing Education*, 48 (1): 17–23.

Parsole, E. and Wray, M. (2000) *Coaching and Mentoring*. London: Kogan Page.

Rose, G.L., Rukstalis, M.R. and Schuckit, M.A. (2005) 'Informal mentoring between faculty and medical students', *Academic Medicine*, 80 (4): 344–8.

key concepts in healthcare education

23 partnership working

Annette Jinks

DEFINITIONS

The areas that are addressed here are notions of partnership working and involvement of stakeholders in educational initiatives. Partnership working refers to relationships formed between individuals or groups that are characterised by mutual cooperation and responsibilities. There are many sorts of partnerships that educationalists need to develop in order to achieve the goals of an educational endeavour. For example, when undertaking curriculum development activities partnership working is important so as to include a range of differing expertise and to ensure that the programme prepares practitioners for the imperatives of clinical practice.

Stakeholders are people or organisations that have a shared interest in an enterprise. Decisions regarding the design, delivery and evaluation of educational programmes or initiatives need to include the perspectives of multiple stakeholders. Stakeholders in any educational endeavour will include people such as programme commissioners and educationalists themselves along with service personnel, users and carers and a range of representatives from pertinent statutory and voluntary agencies.

An initiative that may be instigated by either education or service personnel which epitomises both partnership working and the importance of involving key stakeholders is the development of a Practice Development Unit (PDU). Such units are based in clinical settings and usually focus on developing or enhancing care through education and/or research initiatives. Early forerunners of PDUs were Nursing Development Units (NDU), which as the name implies were nursing orientated. Modern-day PDUs, however, cross professional boundaries with all members of the multi-disciplinary team encouraged to be involved.

Partnership working is inherent in the development of a PDU. For example, a number of Higher Education Institutions (HEIs) have developed criteria and systems for the accreditation of such units. Staff from the HEI and practice staff work closely together to ensure that standards of practice are met in order that the unit may be accredited by the HEI as having PDU status. To achieve the goals set for the PDU, whether they be research or education or a mixture of both, partnership working and the involvement of key stakeholders such the clinical team, educational staff, service and educational managers, and service users and carers is essential.

KEY POINTS

- Partnership working and involvement of key stakeholders are key to the success of all educational initiatives.
- Development of a PDU is an example of how partnership working and stakeholder collaboration are crucial for the success of the unit.
- PDU personnel are drawn from all members of the multi-disciplinary team.
- Some authors relate how PDUs can help reduce the theory–practice divide.
- Some HEIs have developed PDU accreditation systems.
- Action research methods are particularly suited for the practice improvement projects that many PDUs undertake.

DISCUSSION

Partnership working between educationalists and service staff is crucial for a PDU's success. There is, however, little literature that focuses on how such units enhance the relationship between the practice and academia. Happell (2006) does relate that in Melbourne, Australia, a Nursing Clinical Development Unit (NCDU) was introduced which had several aims, one of which was enhancing of the relationship between the clinical field and academia. Underpinning this aim was the desire to reduce the theory–practice divide. Happell conducted a qualitative evaluation with nurses who had participated in the NCDU programme and found that the new relationships that were forged between practice and academia were highly valued by most participants. However, Happell concludes that the extent to which these improved relationship have impacted on the utilisation of research findings by nurses engaged in practice could not be clearly determined.

The problem of the rift between theory and practice is deeply rooted in the history of healthcare education. Discrepancies between what is taught in an academic setting and what is practised in a clinical situation has long been of concern to both educationalists and service staff. Happell (2006) argues that in order for health professionals to acknowledge the value of research to practice and seek to utilise research findings in their practice often requires a significant cultural change. As often in the past, academic researchers have been critical of clinical staff and their lack of interest in, and use of, research, while clinical staff have been critical of researchers whose work is seen as having no practical value. A PDU with an active research programme can help ensure that clinical staff do become at least research aware, if not research active, and that the research conducted is relevant to practice.

Research, whether it is represented by development and use of evidence-based practice guidelines or actually setting up a formalised research programme, is to the fore in many PDU accreditation systems. Action research processes that involve groups of practitioners observing-reflecting-acting-evaluating-modifying on their practice is identified by Jinks and Marsden (2007) as being particularly suitable for PDU work. A powerful and liberating form of professional enquiry concerns practitioners who are supported by educational colleagues in investigating their own practice. A number of authors identify use of action research methodologies as an appropriate model for PDU research activities. For example, Graham (1996) states that action research methods are important if an understanding is to be gained of the importance of nursing practice to patient care. Similarly, Walsh and Walsh (1998) relate that the growth of PDUs will provide many action research opportunities for collaborative ventures involving educationalists and health-care professionals. Bell and Proctor (1998) also describe how nursing, like other healthcare professional groups, has experienced considerable difficulty in implementing research findings derived from conventional approaches to research and this difficulty can be overcome through use of action research approaches.

There are a number of studies that have examined the research activities of P/NDU staff. For example, Bell and Proctor (1998) conducted a study that utilised qualitative research methods and was aimed at eliciting nurses' accounts of their involvement with nursing research and their interpretations of the meaning of these projects for their practice. The findings revealed two types of research activities: one core group of nurses were actively engaged in the research projects whereas the other more peripheral group were involved in data collection. However, this peripheral group were not peripheral to other aspects of practice development initiatives. These nurses often undertook training and development courses that were directly related to the immediate concerns of their everyday practice. So, whilst the data did confirm the development of nursing skills and practice, these were not always related to research activities.

There have been a number of studies that have evaluated the impact and outputs of P/NDUs. For example, Avallone and Gibbon (1998) examined nurses' perceptions of their work environment in a NDU, Bowles and Bowles (2000) investigated clinical leadership issues in NDUs, Pearson (1997) evaluated the King's Fund teams' NDU network and Gerrish (2001) described a pluralistic evaluation of six P/NDUs. Glasper et al. (2000) gave the findings of a quinquennial evaluation of a paediatric outpatients department with King's Fund accreditation, whereas Walsh and Walsh (1998) reported on the findings of a study designed to establish the level and quality of teamwork necessary for successful PDU development. The study of Walsh and Walsh is of particular relevance as it was found that if clinical teams already worked together, this effectively augured well for the eventual success of the PDU.

CASE STUDY

The following case study describes how a Haematology Practice Development Unit (HPDU) was conceived and initiated at a large acute teaching hospital in the North-West of England and how partnership working was central to its success. The HPDU was working towards accreditation status with a local HEI. That the unit demonstrates clinical excellence is a vital component of these accreditation processes. Existing quality systems and reporting mechanisms at the Trust were utilised to establish the area's standards of practice. For example, use of Health Commission standards, clinical governance and performance review reports formed part of an accreditation portfolio that the HPDU team needed to present to the HEI and Trust steering group members in order to gain accreditation. The steering group were the key stakeholders in the development of the PDU and included senior Trust and HEI managers.

The aim of the HPDU, in line with similar PDUs, was to develop and enhance clinical practice over a specified time period of three years. Working with staff from the HEI, HPDU staff were helped to develop plans for a small number of action research projects. These focused on practice improvement and included such things as exploring patients' perceptions of blood transfusion treatment, investigating the interplay between medical, nursing and patient decision making in medical ward rounds and patients' experiences when being treated for lymphatic disorders. In all of these projects there was a direct aim to explore patient perspectives of their care regimes and improve care as a result of new insights. Subsidiary aims of the HPDU related to staff development and enhancing the research capability of nurses working in the unit. For example, planned options for staff undertaking the action research projects included being able to gain academic credit up to, and including, doctoral level of study.

Ensuring the robustness of the HPDU research activities was achieved through the close partnership arrangements set up, involving Trust and HEI personnel. For example, the overall research aims were confirmed during the accreditation processes, which involved senior Trust and university staff. Exact details of project aims, objectives, design and methods were, however, discussed and debated at HPDU operational group meetings. Here practitioners, researchers and educationalists work closely together developing and reflecting on exact project details. When the aims, objectives and project design were generally agreed, individual HPDU researchers leading on a particular project were supported by university staff members to prepare a formal research proposal. Subsequently, the university Faculty Research Committee considers the research proposals and makes recommendations for approval or amendment. Ethical approval for projects is also obtained from the local NHS Ethics Committee and Trust research governance systems.

The systems evolved were therefore very similar to those that university researchers and research degree students undertake when the robustness of their research is considered. The whole process is designed to ensure that clinical and university support and review are married together so that the rigour of the research, research governance and ethical compliance of the proposed research are ensured. Whilst it is a lengthy process it is believed that it gives a sound foundation for the development of the individual projects. Similarly, as each project is rolled out peer and university support is crucial to ensure that the research methods, data collection and analysis approaches are robust.

CONCLUSION

It may be concluded that developing practice so that patients receive optimum care is the main driver for development of PDUs and the various planned action research projects. However, to separate these ideals from aims to contribute to the personal development of staff is difficult. For example, development of the PDU staff research skills and possible educational accreditation of such learning are important elements of the strategies described. Similarly, it is thought that learning experiences for university staff and revitalisation of their practice perceptions will be an important outcome. Partnership working and the involvement of key stakeholders are central to achieving these aims

See also: experiential and work-based learning; research and scholarly activity; service user and carer involvement

FURTHER READING

Day, C., Elliott, J., Somekh, B. and Winter, R. (2002) *Theory and Practice in Action Research*. Oxford: Symposium Books.
Page, S., Allsopp, D. and Cosley, S. (1998) *The Practice Development Unit: An Experiment in Multidisciplinary Innovation*. London: Whurr Publications.

REFERENCES

Avallone, I. and Gibbon, B. (1998) 'Nurses' perceptions of their work environment in a Nursing Development Unit', *Journal of Advanced Nursing*, 27 (6): 1193–201.
Bell, M. and Proctor, S. (1998) 'Developing nurse practitioners to develop practice: the experiences of nurses working on a Nursing Development Unit', *Journal of Nursing Management*, 6 (2): 61–9.
Bowles, A. and Bowles, N.B. (2000) 'A comparative study of transformational leadership in nursing development units and conventional clinical settings', *Journal of Nursing Management*, 8 (2): 69–76.
Gerrish, K. (2001) 'A pluralistic evaluation of nursing/practice development units', *Journal of Clinical Nursing*, 10 (1): 109–18.
Glasper, E.A., Brooking, J. and Rachael, H. (2000) 'Multiprofessional perceptions of a paediatric nursing development unit', *British Journal of Nursing*, 9 (7): 415–22.
Graham, I. (1996) 'A presentation of a conceptual framework and its use in the definition of nursing development within a number of nursing development units', *Journal of Advanced Nursing*, 23 (2): 260–6.

partnership working

Happell, B. (2006) 'Nursing Clinical Development Unit: a strategy to promote the relationship between practice and academia', *International Journal of Psychiatric Nursing Research*, 11 (3): 1319–30.

Jinks, A.M. and Marsden, C. (2007) 'Use of action research in practice development units', *Practice Development in HealthCare*, 6 (3): 165–75.

Pearson, A. (1997) 'An evaluation of King's Fund Centre Nursing Development Unit network 1989–91', *Journal of Clinical Nursing*, 6 (1): 25–33.

Walsh, M. and Walsh, A. (1998) 'Practice development units: a study of teamwork', *Nursing Standard*, 12 (33): 35–8.

24 peer support and observation

Julie Bailey-McHale and Lyz Moore

DEFINITION

Peer support and observation can be defined in a number of ways in healthcare education. It can be a dynamic mode through which students learn from, support and assess each other. Peer support can also be used by lecturers whilst learning the craft of healthcare education and as a method of continually engaging in reflection of their practice as educators. Recently, in Higher Education (HE) peer observation of teaching has become an integral part of the assessment of teaching practice for new lecturers. Within HE there is an expectation that educators will participate in reciprocal peer support and observation as a form of professional development (Quality Assurance Agency (QAA), 2000). Peer observation comes under various guises, including peer observation of learning and teaching (POLT) (Gosling, 2002), peer observation of teachers (POT) (Hammersley-Fletcher and Orsmond, 2004), peer review (Gosling and O'Connor, 2006) and peer teaching-assessment (Trujillo et al., 2009). It has been recognised that peer support and observation should, and can, take place in any learning environment, including face-to-face teaching, blended and e-learning contexts (Bennett and Barp, 2008).

The principles of peer learning are closely linked to andragogy and adult learning (Knowles, 1990). Tennant (1997) argues that a key aspect of adult learning is the establishment of mutual and collaborative learning relationships.

The purpose of these relationships with peers is ultimately to encourage learning and development. It is the considered reflections of those defined as the learners' peers that can enable this to happen.

KEY POINTS

- Learning should be at the heart of peer observation and support.
- Peer support and observation can facilitate critical self-evaluation and assist in identifying professional development needs.
- Although there is an increased use of peer observation within HE Institutions, the use of POT is not without criticism.
- The principles of peer observation and support can be utilised to facilitate learning within student groups by the healthcare educator.

DISCUSSION

Two aspects of peer support and observation will be explored here: firstly its use as a tool to assess the quality of teaching, particularly for new healthcare lecturers, and secondly, the use of peer learning as a teaching method within healthcare education.

Peer Observation of Teaching

Peer support and observation can take place within any mode of educational delivery, including face-to-face, e-learning, blended learning and any combination of teaching contexts. Mutual benefits of peer support and observation have been reported by those observing and by the observed (Kell and Annetts, 2009; Kohut et al., 2007). Peer support and observation can encourage academic discourse using constructive feedback to share areas for development and best practice. The opportunity to facilitate exploration between colleagues allows for mutual development and professional advancement through sharing epistemological ideologies in a reflective way. Teaching, by its very nature, is a public activity and so is open to evaluation and feedback. Critics of peer support and observation suggest the imposition of this system is merely a tick-box approach to evidencing standards (Shortland, 2004). Arguably, the formality of being observed by a colleague can impinge on the autonomy and creativity of the healthcare educator.

A structured approach to POT ensures that some of these criticisms can be addressed. The supportive element within peer observation is a pivotal factor in enhancing the effectiveness of the process, making professional development meaningful. Discussions should focus on affording both educators the opportunity to negotiate ground rules and establish a safe environment, modelled on mutual respect and the anticipation of an equally positive professional development experience. Gosling and O'Connor (2006) suggest the observee should control the focus of the observation, identifying areas of professional development. A written pro forma should remain confidential between the

This pro forma is to be completed by the observee and given to the observer. It should remain confidential between the educators engaged in peer support and observation	
Observee Name	Observer Name
Planned date of observation	Academic level/year
Subject title	Activity (lecture, seminar, tutorial)
Length of session	Number of students
What aspects of student learning would be most interesting for you to explore?	
Is there any aspect of your teaching or assessment practice you would like to change?	
Are there aspects of your teaching that you would like to investigate or reflect on further? (This might be to understand better why something works well as much as something that is not working successfully)	
What are your goals in teaching your subject? Are they being achieved?	
Specific areas of development for observation	
Specific focus/activity to be observed: How does this fit with the module/curriculum?	
Observer Notes	
Aspect of practice selected for focus by observee	Observer's notes and comments
Focus:	
Focus:	

Figure 24.1 Pre-observation pro forma for peer review (adapted from Gosling and O'Connor, 2006)

observee and observer. The role of the observer is to assist the observee to identify the focus of the peer support and observation. The use of a framework to structure the peer support and observation process (Figure 24.1) will encourage both parties to take an objective view, leading to constructive evaluation, feedback, discussion, exploration and reflection, thus reducing anxieties.

The observer can learn as much from observing as the observee can from being observed. Observers can learn from the approaches their colleague takes to structuring learning within their teaching practice and detect alternative methodologies to enhance their own practice. This process of developing collegiate trust through reciprocal collaboration (Martin and Double, 1998) will have the effect of reducing anxieties relating to being observed in the long term, because the observee will at some point become an observer. Thus, the peer support and observation process will be experienced from both perspectives and should evolve to become a mutually beneficial constructive reflection of practice (Kell and Annetts, 2009).

Peer Support and Learning

The principles of peer learning are closely related to a humanistic approach to learning and teaching and the principles of andragogy. Peer learning can happen in both informal and formal settings and occurs when students learn from and with each other (Boud et al., 2001). Topping (2005) goes further and suggests that peer learning involves people from similar social groupings, who are not professional teachers, helping each other to learn. Learning through shared discovery is important and educators should be aware of the potential power of this type of activity. The work by humanist theorists is important here in emphasising the characteristics of an effective educator using this type of approach. Crucially, the educator should be genuine, self-aware and trust the feelings and views of the learner.

Peer assessment can also be a useful strategy to facilitate deeper learning as it involves students assessing the quality of each other's work, either written or skills-based (van den Berg et al., 2006). Feedback is an essential component of any assessment strategy and the students giving feedback benefit from this activity as much as students receiving the feedback. This reflects the comments made earlier regarding POT and the reported benefits to the educator giving the feedback. Quinn and Hughes (2007) describe some of the potential problems with peer assessment, including student collusion and the desire to say only positive things. One resolution to this is to use only peer assessment in a formative manner, however this can encourage the students to regard the assessment as less important than others.

CASE STUDY

Aalin has recently been appointed as a lecturer in nursing at a local university. She has 15 years' experience working as a community nurse. She has always been interested in education and was a mentor in the practice setting. She regularly taught in the university on her specialist subject. This change in career has left Aalin feeling de-skilled and a novice once again. Aalin has commenced a Postgraduate Certificate in Education. A key element of the programme is formative assessment of her teaching practice by a peer, followed by summative assessment by the programme leader. Aalin's first teaching assessment was quite rushed and she did not get the opportunity to speak to her assessor beforehand. It had not been clear which specific elements of Aalin's teaching assessment her peer should review. Consequently, Aalin received general feedback that was not explicit enough for her to reflect upon and develop in her teaching. This experience left Aalin questioning the benefits of peer review, which she discussed with her mentor. They agreed an action plan which included formally planning the peer review process. Aalin led this process by identifying her objectives with her chosen peer reviewer, including how she negotiated shared outcomes for the session with the student group and how she encouraged group interaction. The second teaching assessment went really well and Aalin benefited from the focused feedback of her reviewer. The reviewer also commented on the benefits of being a reviewer and learning from observing Aalin. This positive planned review encouraged Aalin to reflect upon the potential benefits of peer learning that could be adapted for her own student group. Aalin planned a number of teaching sessions in the forthcoming semester which included problem-based learning incorporating the principle of students learning from each other. Aalin also introduced the concept of formative peer assessment of skills. Aalin emphasised the importance of planning the review experience with her peers and students, and continues to use peer support and observation to reflect on and enhance her professional practice and that of her students.

CONCLUSION

The principles of peer support and observation are essential components of any healthcare educator's range of strategies. There are challenges associated with both peer observation of teaching and aspects of peer learning. However, the benefits of both can be significant and so are an essential part of healthcare education.

See also: academic staff development; assessment; e-learning; humanist learning theories

FURTHER READING

Blakemore, J. (2005) 'A critical evaluation of peer review via teaching observation within higher education', *International Journal of Educational Management*, 19 (3): 218–32.
Carter, V. (2008) 'Five steps to becoming a better peer reviewer', *College Teaching*, 56 (2): 85–8.

REFERENCES

Bennett, S. and Barp, D. (2008) 'Peer observation – a case for doing it online', *Teaching in Higher Education*, 13 (5): 559–70.
Boud, D., Cohen, R. and Sampson, J. (2001) *Peer Learning in Higher Education: Learning from and with Each Other*. London: Kogan Page.
Gosling, D. (2002) 'Models of peer observation of teaching'. Retrieved from LTSN website: www.ltsn.ac.uk/genericcentre
Gosling, D. and O'Connor, K. (2006) 'From peer observation of teaching to review of professional practice (RPP): a model for Continuing Professional Development', *Educational Developments*, 7 (3): 1–4.
Hammersley-Fletcher, L. and Ormond, P. (2004) 'Evaluating our peers: is peer observation a meaningful process?', *Studies in Higher Education*, 29 (4): 489–503.
Kell, C. and Annetts, S. (2009) 'Peer review of teaching embedded practice or policy-holding complacency?', *Innovations in Education and Teaching International*, 46 (1): 61–70.
Kohut, G., Burnap, C. and Yon, M. (2007) 'Peer observation of teaching: perceptions of the observer and the observed', *College Teaching*, 55 (1): 19–25.
Knowles, M. (1990) *The Adult Learner: A Neglected Species*, 4th edn. Houston, TX: Gulf.
Martin, G. and Double, J. (1998) 'Developing Higher Education teaching skills through peer observation and collaborative reflection', *Innovations in Teaching and Training Interactions*, 35: 161–70.
Quality Assurance Agency (2000) *Handbook for Academic Review*. London: QAA.
Quinn, F. and Hughes, S.J. (2007) *Quinn's Principles and Practice of Nurse Education*, 5th edn. Cheltenham: Nelson Thornes.

key concepts in
healthcare education

Shortland, S. (2004) 'Peer observation: a tool for staff development or compliance?', *Journal of Further and Higher Education*, 28 (2): 219–28.

Tennant, M. (1997) *Psychology and Adult Learning*, 2nd edn. London: Routledge.

Topping, K. (2005) 'Trends in peer learning', *Educational Psychology*, 25 (6): 631–45.

Trujillo, J., DiVall, M.V., Barr, J., Gonyeau, M., Van Amburgh, J.A., Matthews, S.J. and Qualters, D. (2009) 'Development of a peer teaching-assessment program and a peer observation and evaluation tool', *American Journal of Pharmaceutical Education*, 72 (6): 1–9.

van den Berg, I., Admiraal, W. and Pilot, A. (2006) 'Design principles and outcomes of peer assessment in Higher Education', *Studies in Higher Education*, 31 (3): 341–56.

25 practice teaching

Karen Holland

DEFINITION

Practice teaching is, in principle, teaching in the situational context of a practice environment. In healthcare this could encompass a myriad of work contexts where students and practitioners are either taught, or themselves teach others.

KEY POINTS

- Practice teaching is context-specific.
- It requires consideration of the focus of healthcare, e.g. patients.
- It must be viewed in relation to the culture of a working healthcare environment or a community of practice.

DISCUSSION

Teaching cannot be viewed in isolation from learning, given that for teaching to be effective in any context one must know and understand how students learn. In addition, for teaching in practice to be effective there is a need to be familiar with, and understand, the practice environment in its broadest sense and, for some teachers, their individual practice situation. Walker et al. point out that 'teaching approaches that facilitate adult learning are critical in supporting students to transfer their learning into practice and in developing their learning in practice' (2008: 60). Many practitioners are involved in teaching

(Jarvis and Gibson [1997] refer to practitioner teachers), but this is not normally their primary function. The role that teachers working in Higher Education have in a practice context has long been an issue of debate and contention. For some, a joint role became possible in lecturer–practitioner posts, but in the main they have adopted a link teacher role. Another role with significant teaching responsibility in practice is that of the mentor, especially in nursing and midwifery (Nursing and Midwifery Council, 2008). However, the mentor has become a 'catch-all' role for teaching, assessing and facilitating learning in relation to integration of theory and practice. This is at the same time as being employed to undertake the role as a professional practitioner and expected to fulfil the obligations inherent in it.

A key role, which still exists in countries such as Australia, was that of the clinical teacher, who was tasked with teaching the art and science of professional nursing in the practice arena or clinical practicum. According to Malik and Aston, practice teaching is very different from classroom teaching: 'it is unpredictable, emotional, seldom static and creates unique challenges for the individual teacher' (2003: 135). This requires that a practice teacher not only has teaching skills and knowledge of the learner and learning, but also critical decision making and clinical reasoning skills. Even students can be involved in teaching their peers as part of their learning experience in practice and during their programmes of study are required to engage in learning about their own and others' learning styles and how to undertake a teaching session. A more recent development in a practice setting has been the introduction of the patient or service user as teacher (Stockhausen, 2008).

For healthcare educators, or practice teachers, the most important aspect of their role is to create a link for the student between theory and practice experience and one way of enabling this is through what Schon (1983) defined as reflective practice. To enable and facilitate reflective practice in learners, teachers need to be reflective practitioners themselves. To do this effectively they need to demonstrate that their practice is evidence-based and ensure that time is built in to reflect on their actions in order to learn from them. In turn, this can then be used to develop skills in learners, in order for them to progress from novice practitioners who may think in 'steps' to more experienced practitioners who think in 'wholes'. Using learning theories that facilitate this process can help teachers to stage their teaching sessions or experiences, which in turn will help them in their assessment of learning. One of the most important ways of learning in practice is through observing others and then copying what they do or how they do it; this is often known as role modelling (Bandura, 1986). Lave and Wenger (1991) call this learning from experts in a specific context *situated learning*, which happens over a period of time.

Making a decision on which theoretical framework to use will in part be dependent on what is to be taught or learnt. For example, consider the giving of medication. Once the basic principles are grasped students will need to understand situations where decisions are not clear and where they have to consider various options. Here the learner becomes an active participant in the learning situation, and feedback becomes more interactive. If it is clear that this learning helps students to 'fit in' with others, the students are praised for doing well. This will then reinforce a positive learning experience. This type of learning within a specific social context is known as a *social learning theory* (Bandura, 1986).

Walker et al. (2008) set out a number of different teaching methods that can be used with learners in practice. These include: discussion; presentation on a specific topic; reading and questioning; investigating or researching a topic related to practice; observing and reflecting. Many of these are essential in the use of problem-based or enquiry-based learning in practice.

CASE STUDY

Problem-based learning (PBL) is well established in healthcare education, in particular within the education setting, but in practice this is not as well defined (Ehrenberg and Haggblom, 2007). For our purposes here we will focus on an interprofessional group of learners in a unit for patients who have experienced a stroke. This scenario had been utilised previously in the safe environment of a student seminar exploring integrated care service delivery and had been evaluated as a positive learning experience by the students (Holland et al., 2006).

The principles of PBL involve the practice teacher acting as facilitator of learning rather than as a teacher, and who sets the scene by providing the students with a 'set problem' to explore. In PBL the students 'learn to be self-directed, independent and inter-dependent learners motivated to solve a problem' (Kiley et al., 2000: 3).

The Scenario and PBL trigger

What are the roles of each of the health and social care professionals caring for the patients in this stroke unit and how do they contribute to the progress and care of the patients? (The problem in this situation is to gain a collective understanding of multi-disciplinary working in caring for a patient who has experienced a stroke.)

The PBL learning experience

The basic principles of PBL that the students have to manage in this scenario are: agree on a way of working together and individually, identify what they know or don't know already, gather information from a variety of resources and share it with the group. Following this, they might decide to undertake further searching for information prior to presenting their experiences and findings, which may involve a number of meetings. Resources may well involve talking to patients and their families about their experiences of how different professional groups work with them to support their progress. This would of course be undertaken with the support of their supervisors/teachers in practice.

The role of the teacher

The teacher in this learning experience becomes the facilitator and encourages the students to take responsibility for their own learning needs. It is important, however, that in setting a PBL scenario as the teaching method, the teacher does not abandon the students to their own devices, but sets up a learning group scenario, interacts with the students and facilitates their learning. The teacher does not normally provide information for the students, but is there to stimulate discussion and learning in the group. The teacher may also intervene and help the students to work out particularly difficult tasks or group dynamics. Gaining these skills is essential to being able to implement PBL as a teaching method in practice.

One of the most important aspects of this method of teaching or facilitating learning in practice is to anticipate the outcomes or learning goals for the PBL experience (in other words, what you want the students to have achieved, which may or may not be shared with them) and, most importantly, the assessment of student learning and the impact on patient care. Ensuring the students have access to resources either in the practice environment or elsewhere is also vital. The added value of the practice teacher role in PBL is to act as a positive role model for the learners, who are encouraged to value their contribution to the experience of the group.

The case study outcomes

The students will need to learn the role of each health and social care professional involved in the care of the stroke unit patients and the reason for their involvement. This information may arise from interviewing each other or qualified personnel. The students can be encouraged to keep a reflective journal of their findings and thoughts on their learning experience whilst in this placement. They may have also undertaken literature searching in the library and obtained articles about the various roles to bring back to discuss in the group. Collating the information into a package to leave in the practice area for other students and staff to read could also be a positive outcome. Talking to patients and their families would normally be undertaken as part of the students' learning experience in practice and would be added to by learning about how they are experiencing their illness and being a patient on the unit. Students need to be given feedback as they discuss their findings, and for this exercise it would be formative. The practice teacher may also add his or her own assessment of learning through a 'Unit Quiz' about the various roles generally and how they are involved specifically in the care of the patients.

Telling feedback comments received by Holland et al. from the students involved in this study included: 'if we don't understand each other's roles, how do we expect the patient to do so?' and 'if they come into a Health Centre and are faced with lots of different professions looking after them, how do they know who does what in their care?' (2006: 47). An outcome of this exercise could be a small pamphlet for patients and their relatives of the various personnel in the unit and an explanation of the role they play in patient care.

CONCLUSION

Supporting the transfer of learning to a wide range of practice situations is an essential criterion of practice teaching. Professional practice relies on practitioners who become effective, positive role models for learners in environments that should, in turn, be effective communities of learning.

See also: behavioural learning theories; cognitive learning theories; experiential and work-based learning; humanist learning theories; problem-based learning; reflection; teaching styles; transformative learning

FURTHER READING

Glen, S. and Parker, P. (2003) *Supporting Learning in Nursing Practice.* Basingstoke: Palgrave Macmillan.
Walker, J., Crawford, K. and Parker, J. (2008) *Practice Education in Social Work: A Handbook for Practice Teachers, Assessors and Educators.* Exeter: Learning Matters.

REFERENCES

Bandura, A. (1986) *Social Foundations of Thought and Action: A Social Cognitive Theory.* Englewood Cliffs, NJ: Prentice-Hall.
Ehrenberg, A.C. and Haggblom, M. (2007) 'Problem-based learning in clinical nursing education: integrating theory and practice', *Nurse Education in Practice*, 7 (2): 67–74.
Holland, K., Warne, T. and Lawrence, K. (2006) *Shaping the Future for Primary Care Education and Training Project: Finding the Evidence for Education and Training to Deliver Integrated Health and Social Care: The Project Experience.* Salford: University of Salford.
Jarvis, P. and Gibson, S. (1997) *The Teacher Practitioner and Mentor in Nursing, Midwifery, Health Visiting and the Social Services.* Cheltenham: Stanley Thornes.
Kiley, M., Mullins, G., Peterson, R. and Rogers, T. (2000) *Leap into ... Problem-based Learning.* Retrieved from the University of Adelaide, Centre for Learning and Professional Development website: www.adelaide.edu.au/clpd/.../leap/leapinto/ProblemBased Learning.pdf
Lave, J. and Wenger, E. (1991) *Situated Learning: Legitimate Peripheral Participation.* Cambridge: Cambridge University Press.
Malik, M. and Aston, L. (2003) 'Providing educator support for practice learning', in S. Glen and P. Parker (eds), *Supporting Learning in Nursing Practice.* Basingstoke: Palgrave Macmillan. pp. 126–50.
Nursing and Midwifery Council (2008) *Standards to Support Learning and Assessment in Practice.* London: NMC.
Schon, D.A. (1983) *The Reflective Practitioner.* Aldershot: Avebury.
Stockhausen, L.J. (2008) 'The patient as experience broker in clinical learning', *Nurse Education in Practice*, 9 (3): 184–9.
Walker, J., Crawford, K. and Parker, J. (2008) *Practice Education in Social Work: A Handbook for Practice Teachers, Assessors and Educators.* Exeter: Learning Matters.

practice teaching

26 problem-based learning

Jean Mannix and Annette McIntosh

DEFINITION

Problem-based learning (PBL), as the name suggests, can be simply defined as using problems as the basis for students' learning. More specifically, PBL is a process involving an andragogical approach to education. In essence, PBL seeks to place the student at the heart of an active learning experience, gaining a deeper understanding and internalisation of knowledge by working through, and solving, problems. Within this experiential process, skills such as critical thinking and reflection are fostered. In implementing a PBL strategy, some Higher Education Institutions have used terms such as enquiry- or case-based learning. However, as Wilkie and Burns (2003) note, it is often the case that the principles of these strategies are not fully in line with the PBL philosophy and are based on other approaches such as discovery or problem-solving learning.

KEY POINTS

- PBL is an educational process in which students take control of their own learning, facilitated by lecturing staff and the use of well constructed, realistic problems.
- PBL is a strategy that promotes the development of critical thinking, analysis and reflection, alongside teamworking and collaboration.
- There are challenges associated with PBL, including resource implications and the preparation of staff and students.

DISCUSSION

PBL developed within medical education in the 1960s (Barrows and Tamblyn, 1980) and was also originally used as a curriculum approach in Australian nurse education in the early 1990s (Creedy et al., 1992), before being widely adopted as a learning strategy within health education (Barrow et al., 2002; Wilkie and Burns, 2003). Barrows (1996) described six core characteristics of PBL in his model:

- Learning is student-centred.
- Students work in small groups.
- Lecturers are facilitators and guides.
- Authentic problems are presented prior to any study of the area.
- Problems are used as tools to achieve the knowledge and skills to solve the problems.
- New information is acquired through self-directed learning.

In addition, as Dochy et al. (2003) noted, a generally agreed supplementary characteristic is that of an assessment process that takes into account the PBL approach. The successful use of PBL has both advantages and challenges.

Advantages of PBL

PBL has long been recognised as a strategy that encourages students to work collaboratively (Maudsley and Strivens, 2000), a crucial element in professional education. The key advantages that emerge from using a PBL approach are shared learning, collaborative working and development of problem solving and critical thinking skills (Bechtel et al., 1999). To prepare healthcare professionals for the unpredictable context of clinical practice, PBL provides a dynamic and relevant learning experience for students to take risks, try out ideas, think independently and be more self-directed (Gidman and Mannix, 2007). It has been noted that PBL has the potential to foster the necessary learning environment required for professional education (Carey and Whittaker, 2002; Wilkie and Burns, 2003). It emphasises problem solving in real world practice, encouraging students to explore and find solutions within a safe environment and develop a greater understanding and insight into practice (Gidman and Mannix, 2007). This approach to learning provides the opportunity for students to deconstruct ideas through the processes inherent in PBL, thus enabling the generation of innovative practice.

Adopting a PBL approach may well render the learning more relevant and challenging, both to students and to lecturers, thus increasing motivation. Healthcare professionals need to be equipped with critical thinking skills and to become self directed, lifelong learners. It is argued, therefore, that traditional methods of teaching need to be redesigned to support professional development within the competences required for working in the clinical environment (Bechtel et al., 1999; Wilkie and Burns, 2003). Gidman and Mannix (2007) opined that PBL is an innovative strategy that may help bridge the theory–practice gap, reducing the inconsistency between what is taught in the classroom and what students experience in practice. Interprofessional practice is another essential component for professional education. PBL can be used to promote interprofessional learning, equipping students for real world practice and encouraging the contextualisation of tangible scenarios that are realistic and firmly rooted in practice.

Overall, PBL has many advantages. It can aid students to gain confidence in many areas of practice such as interprofessional working, collaboration, teamwork and interpersonal skills. This evolves through the dynamics of group work, one of the foundations of the PBL strategy. Other essential areas that are enhanced by PBL are the higher-level skills of problem skills, critical thinking and decision making.

Challenges of PBL

As PBL involves the use of an andragogical approach, educators have to be comfortable with, and skilled in, adopting a facilitative, student-centred stance. This requires lecturers to have a commitment to PBL, to accept the role of facilitator and to promote the ethos of the approach to students. The challenge here for some lecturers is that they may be unfamiliar with, or unskilled in, the use of PBL or, as Wilkie and Burns (2003) noted, have a fear of undermining their status and their expertise as teacher and subject expert. The preparation and support of lecturers is therefore necessary to ensure positive learning experiences for the students, including the use of well-designed problems or scenarios. Equally, the students themselves need to be prepared to commit to the ethos of PBL, including taking full responsibility for their own learning (Dolmans et al., 2005; Wilkie and Burns, 2003).

Achieving an effective balance between the level of participation and facilitation involved in PBL is essential and can be challenging for both lecturing staff and students. Dolmans et al. (2005) reported that either too much or too little participation by lecturing staff can lead to problems such as dysfunctional group working and lack of student motivation and commitment.

On an organisational level, there are many potentially problematic aspects involved in PBL. In order to facilitate the small groups, extensive educational resources are required, including classroom space and appropriate numbers of experienced staff. This can be costly, especially when dealing with large student numbers and compared to more traditional teaching methods. In addition, the curriculum needs to be clearly structured to facilitate PBL and to ensure that the pace of the learning is appropriate and clearly communicated to students. Another key challenge is the appropriate design of the problems or scenarios used in the PBL process. These consist of two elements: a trigger that starts the PBL process and a description of the situation or context within which the students will explore the problem. As Dolmans et al. (2005) noted, problems that are too structured or too simple may inhibit the learning process. Rather, what are required are problems that, while realistic, are complex, open-ended and relevant to practice.

The design and use of assessments that acknowledge the PBL process is a further challenge. Dochy et al. (2003) stated that central to this is assessing the application of knowledge in problem-solving and that an important requirement in this respect is to use common and significant problems.

There has been debate about the depth and breadth of knowledge and skills attained by students using a PBL approach compared to students learning through more traditional methods. A meta-analysis of empirically based studies by Dochy et al. (2003) concluded that in relation to the acquisition of skills, defined as the application of knowledge, the use of PBL produced a robustly positive effect, while there was no such effect on the acquisition of knowledge. However, Dochy et al. (2003) noted that while students using a PBL approach may gain slightly less knowledge, more of this is remembered and retained. Albanese (2000) opined that while the effect of PBL on knowledge and skills may be debatable, it is evident that students and staff alike enjoy PBL and the positive effect on the learning environment in itself rendered PBL a worthwhile process.

CASE STUDY

Carol is a new lecturer teaching within an undergraduate programme and is keen to use the PBL strategy. Wai, an experienced Senior Lecturer, suggests that Carol uses scenarios with limited guidance and very little background information. Carol feels that this may not give the students the information they require for an effective learning session. Wai tries to reassure Carol, suggesting that 'letting go' will empower the students and develop the autonomy of the learning event. Carol decides to give the students a scenario with very explicit guidelines and an underpinning bio-psycho-social framework. Following student evaluations, the students indicate that they feel they have acquired a good level of knowledge and understanding, were well supported and stayed within their comfort zone. Carol later reflects upon these comments and decides that in the future she wishes to challenge the students. During the next session the students are given a limited scenario and PBL artefacts. At the beginning the students constantly seek reassurance and guidance in generating their learning needs and exploring and solving the elements within the scenario. However, Carol acts as a facilitator and guide, not as a teacher. This is an uncomfortable experience for both Carol and the students. However, the students' learning from the session exceeds Carol's expectations and the students reported that they were challenged, empowered and felt that they had developed their critical thinking, whilst giving consideration to the wider issues.

CONCLUSION

PBL is an andragogical strategy increasingly being employed in the education of healthcare professionals. There are challenges associated with the use of PBL, not least the commitment and preparation of educators and students. However, PBL has many advantages, including the fostering of an ethos of lifelong, student-centred learning and the development of critical thinking and reflective skills. Learning in groups encourages teamworking and collaboration, while the use of realistic problems helps students to explore and contextualise practice-based elements. As such, it can be seen to be a relevant and valuable strategy for use in the preparation of professionals in healthcare.

See also: humanist learning theories; reflection; teaching strategies; teaching styles

FURTHER READING

Wilkie, K. and Burns, I. (2003) *Problem-Based Learning: A Handbook for Nurses*. London: Palgrave.

REFERENCES

Albanese, M. (2000) 'Problem-based learning: why curricula are likely to show little effect on knowledge and clinical skills', *Medical Education*, 34: 729–38.

Barrow, E.J., Lyte, G. and Butterworth, T. (2002) 'An evaluation of problem-based learning in a nursing theory and practice module', *Nurse Education in Practice*, 2 (1): 55–62.

Barrows, H.S. (1996) 'Problem-based learning in medicine and beyond: a brief overview', in L. Wilkerson and W.H Gijselaers (eds), *New Directions for Teaching and Learning*. San Francisco, CA: Jossey–Bass. pp. 3–11.

Barrows, H.S. and Tamblyn, R.M. (1980) *Problem-Based Learning: An Approach to Medical Education*. New York: Springer.

Bechtel, G.A., Davidhizar, R. and Bradshaw, M. (1999) 'Problem based learning in a competency based world', *Nurse Education Today*, 19: 182–7.

Carey, L. and Whittaker, K.A. (2002) 'Experiences of problem based learning: issues for community specialist practitioners', *Nurse Education Today*, 22 (8): 661–7.

Creedy, D., Horsfall, J. and Hand, B. (1992) 'Problem-based learning in nurse education: an Australian view', *Journal of Advanced Nursing*, 17 (6): 727–33.

Dochy, F., Segers, M., van den Bossche, P. and Gijbels, D. (2003) 'Effects of problem-based learning: a meta-analysis', *Learning and Instruction*, 13: 533–68.

Dolmans, D.H.J.M., de Grave, W., Wolfhagen, I.H.A.P. and van der Vleuten, C.P.M. (2005) 'Problem-based learning: future challenges for educational practice and research', *Medical Education*, 39: 732–41.

Gidman, J. and Mannix, J. (2007) 'Problem based learning', in J. Woodhouse (ed.), *Strategies for Healthcare Education: How to Teach in the 21st Century*. Oxford: Radcliffe. pp. 29–41.

Maudsley, G. and Strivens, J. (2000) 'Promoting professional knowledge, experiential learning and critical thinking for medical students', *Medical Education*, 34: 535–44.

Wilkie, K. and Burns, I. (2003) *Problem-Based learning: A Handbook for Nurses*. London: Palgrave.

27 professional accountability

Elisabeth Clark and Chris Cox

DEFINITION

Accountability means being answerable for one's decisions and actions, and being answerable requires being able to explain and justify a decision when called upon to do so (that is, giving an account of one's actions). There are different types of accountability. There is *professional accountability*, whereby healthcare practitioners are accountable to their statutory bodies, for example the Chartered Society of Physiotherapy (CSP) or the Nursing and Midwifery Council (NMC). Being *personally accountable* involves the interaction between the professional and the patient/client, who can bring a civil claim that may result in a finding of negligence against the professional and payment of compensation. Professional educators are *contractually accountable* to their employer for their actions, their use of resources and the reputation of the organization, which can lead to disciplinary action and, possibly, dismissal for a breach of contract. In addition, healthcare professionals are *accountable to society* and this may lead to a criminal prosecution for a criminal offence, with the sanction of a fine or even imprisonment.

We focus here on professional and personal accountability, which embraces all of the healthcare professions. Although there are variations in emphasis between the professions, the underlying principles of professional accountability are essentially very similar.

KEY POINTS

- Whenever a healthcare professional exercises their professional judgement and skills on a patient's/client's behalf, the individual owes the patient a professional and legal duty of care.
- The public generally assume that all those involved with their care have the necessary qualifications, knowledge, skills, experience, competence and authority to carry out the task when working without direct supervision.
- Professional decisions are subject to scrutiny and the requisite standards of care are determined by the best available evidence, best practice and national

guidelines developed by organisations such as the NHS National Institute for Health and Clinical Excellence (NICE).

- Educators in healthcare have a vital role in facilitating students to develop sound professional knowledge and values, including 'whistle-blowing', that are rooted within professional codes of practice.

DISCUSSION

Evidence shows that there is an identified lack of insight into accountability by professionals in healthcare (NMC, 2008) and that there is a danger that those professionals who are unaware of their accountability may be influenced by unsafe practices (Gould, 2009). For educators in healthcare, there is a need to ensure that students are fully cognisant of the following aspects of professional and personal accountability.

Students

Pre-qualifying students in healthcare must act in a patient's best interests, upholding the reputation of their profession and being guided by their code of practice. Since students are not registered, they cannot be struck off the professional register for failing to follow their code.

Inexperience

The required standard of practice is generally determined by the task rather than the seniority or status of the person carrying it out and it is generally irrelevant who is doing it. What is crucial is that the person is competent to carry out the task safely. A job title does not indicate what an individual is permitted to do in legal terms, so it cannot be assumed, for example, that only doctors can do X, nurses can do Y and healthcare assistants can do Z. The exception arises when statute prescribes who may undertake a particular task, such as the prescribing of controlled drugs, or the compulsory admission or treatment of certain individuals under mental health legislation.

Inexperience can never be used as a defence if there is an issue about professional negligence. If any healthcare worker is uncertain about their competence, they should either not perform the task or carry it out only under proper supervision and support.

Keeping up to date

Health professionals are charged with maintaining a high standard of care at all times and are expected to keep up to date in their field of practice. However, the legal and professional requirement is that an individual's practice reflects what would be acceptable to a responsible and reasonable body of relevant professional opinion; so as long as an individual is acting in accordance with common practice, the fact that he or she has not read every article published in that field of practice does not imply negligence. It is legitimate for a professional to do something that is a deviation from standard practice, but only if the individual concerned is competent and can justify his or her action on the basis of sound evidence and/or demonstrate it was something that another equally competent professional would have done in the same situation.

Employers determine the activities that individual practitioners are permitted to carry out and may restrict what individuals can do, even if they are competent to do it. In this situation practitioners must undertake only those activities permitted by their employer.

Delegation

Effective delegation is a crucial element of professional accountability because the professional who delegates an aspect of care is accountable for the appropriateness of the delegation, which must always be in the best interests of the person being cared for. Any decision to delegate should be based on an assessment of the individual needs of the patient/client and must never compromise existing care. An activity should always be delegated with adequate instructions. It is essential for delegators to satisfy themselves that the individual to whom the task is being delegated fully understands the nature of the delegated task, what is required of them and is competent to carry out the instructions safely and effectively (NMC, 2008). This involves verifying that the person has a qualification that demonstrates they have the necessary skill, checking that they can perform the task competently or teaching them to perform the task. This means that delegators should only delegate tasks that they are competent to perform themselves. In addition, the individual delegating the task is responsible for ensuring that the person is appropriately supervised and supported if necessary. As a further safeguard, the person to whom the task has been delegated must fully understand the scope of the delegated work and their own limitations, and seek advice and assistance from a more experienced colleague if they are uncertain about what to do. The person, i.e. the delegatee, must understand that he or she is legally accountable for their actions. In a dynamic and unpredictable healthcare environment the circumstances within which the task has been delegated may change, making it no longer appropriate to proceed. It is important to provide clear instructions as to whom to inform if a patient's condition changes. This is particularly important in community settings, including people's homes, where the majority of care is unsupervised.

In addition, the person who is delegating is responsible for evaluating whether to continue to delegate the activity after reassessing: (a) the situation at appropriate intervals to ensure that it has not changed; (b) the continuing competence of the person to whom an aspect of care has been delegated; and (c) whether the on-going support arrangements are appropriate.

It is essential that anyone delegating care or undertaking a delegated task is operating within a robust local employment framework that protects the public and ensures safe practice. Once an aspect of care has been delegated to another person, then that person is responsible to his/her line manager for the performance of the delegated activity. The name of the person to whom a task has been delegated should always be clearly stated in patient records (for example, a care plan or patient-held record). The professional is responsible for ensuring that any delegated aspect of care is fully documented by the individual who actually delivers the care.

Professional practitioners can refuse to delegate an activity if they believe that it would be unsafe to do so, or if the person to whom the task would be delegated is not competent to carry it out, or if there is inadequate support and supervision for the individual who would undertake the delegated activity. No healthcare practitioner should be pressurised into delegating a task or accepting a delegated task. In such a situation advice should be sought from the line manager and, if necessary, from the practitioner's professional body. Some professions only allow delegation of duties to members within their profession. For example, midwives are only permitted to delegate their statutory duties to other registered midwives (who have notified their intention to practise to the Local Supervisory Authority and have met all the updating requirements for their midwifery practice) or to a registered medical practitioner (NMC, 2004).

Record keeping

Good record keeping is essential for the delivery of safe and effective care and is therefore a crucial aspect of professional accountability. Patient records must always be stored securely and every member of the healthcare team needs to be aware of the legal requirements and guidance regarding confidentiality, and local practice should reflect local and national policy.

Effective record keeping provides documentary evidence of the services delivered and can improve accountability by demonstrating how decisions relating to patient care were made.

Records must be legible, factual and should not include unnecessary abbreviations. Every entry should include a date and time and be signed (with the person's name and job title printed beside the first entry). Any entry in a patient's electronic record must be attributable to the individual who has written it. No record should ever be falsified, altered after the event or destroyed (unless the individual is authorised to do so). Contemporaneous records are the only accurate and reliable way of documenting care, so records should always be made as soon as possible. Accurate records are crucial when dealing with a complaint or legal investigation. A failure to document care will often mean that alleged negligent care cannot be legally or professionally defended.

Whistle-blowing

Whistle-blowing enables an individual to raise confidentially any significant concerns about the environment of care, including persistent low staffing levels, poor infection control and incompetent professional practice, that militate against safe standards of care and put people at risk of harm or injury (Vinten and Gavin, 2005). This should be done internally within an organisation in the first instance and, only in exceptional circumstances, externally in accordance with relevant legislation, employment policies and good practice. There has been a huge change in the public sector over recent years, and, as part of their accountability, healthcare practitioners have a professional duty to alert the appropriate authorities if another person's fitness to practise or competence is questionable, if their performance is in any way deficient, or if a health professional is prevented from working within their professional code of practice or other nationally agreed standards of care. There can be conflict between a person's responsibilities and duties under their professional code of practice and their employer's interpretation of what is expected under the employment contract. However, it is now recommended that the duty to report professional deficiency is written into employer's terms and conditions of service, thereby protecting whistle-blowers who use appropriate channels to register their concerns.

CASE STUDY

A second-year student nurse is undertaking a placement on a day case unit where children are regularly admitted for surgery. None of the registered nurses working on the unit is a qualified children's nurses. The student is concerned to hear that parents are being advised to fast their child from midnight prior to surgery and knows that this is an outdated practice. She witnesses a registered nurse giving this outdated fasting advice to parents (Morris, 2004).

What should this student do to support safe, evidence-based practice? The student has identified a practice that is not in the children's best interests and is potentially dangerous. If the student remains silent to avoid upsetting a colleague and the possible negative effect on her placement experience, she would not be adhering to the principles of the NMC Code (2008),which require her to work with others to protect and promote the health and wellbeing of patients/clients and to act with integrity. Since health professionals are expected to work effectively as part of a team and share skills and experience for colleagues' benefit, it would be appropriate for the student to discuss her knowledge and the relevant evidence base with the registered nurse. If it were to become apparent that the registered nurse is aware of the evidence and/or the local protocol and is disregarding them, the student has no option but to pursue the uncomfortable route of challenging the practice of a registered nurse. The registered nurse should listen to the student nurse, who is using her recent knowledge to help a colleague keep up to date. The Code expects registered nurses to work cooperatively within teams and respect the skills, expertise and contributions of colleagues alongside facilitating students and others to develop their competence; this includes a student's confidence to challenge practice and speak out when the quality of care is at risk.

CONCLUSION

Healthcare practitioners have a professional and legal duty of care to patients and clients. This involves having the necessary qualifications, knowledge and skills to carry out, or delegate, healthcare practice, including record keeping, and to identify and tackle any significant concerns about standards of care.

Healthcare educators thus have a responsibility to ensure that students develop and maintain the professional knowledge and values embedded within their professional code of practice.

See also: clinical competence; dealing with failing and problem students; quality assurance and enhancement; student support

FURTHER READING

Dimond, B. (2008) *Legal Aspects of Nursing*, 5th edn. Harlow: Pearson Education.
Royal College of Nursing (2008) *Principles to Inform Decision Making: What do I need to know?*, 2nd edn. London: RCN.

REFERENCES

Gould, D. (2009) 'Re-engaging with accountability', *British Journal of Midwifery*, 17 (1): 6.
Morris, R. (2004) 'Speak out or shut up? Accountability and the student nurse', *Paediatric Nursing*, 16 (6): 20 –2.
Nursing and Midwifery Council (2004) *Guidance on Provision of Midwifery Care and Delegation of Midwifery Care to Others*. NMC Circular 1/2004. London: NMC.
Nursing and Midwifery Council (2008) *Supervision, Support and Safety: Analysis of the 2007–08 Local Supervisory Authority Annual Reports to the NMC*. London: NMC.
Vinten, G. and Gavin, T.A. (2005) 'Whistle blowing on health, welfare and safety: the UK experience', *Journal of the Royal Society for the Promotion of Health*, 125 (1): 23–9.

key concepts in
healthcare education

28 quality assurance and enhancement

Jane Fox

Quality isn't something you lay on top of subjects and objects like tinsel on a Christmas tree. Real quality must be the source of the subject and objects, the cone from which the tree must start. (Pirsig, 1999: 292)

DEFINITION

Pirsig (1999) highlights the importance of quality to general life. However, in a public services context, quality has particular meanings and significance. Stoddart (2004) suggests quality is intrinsic to Higher Education (HE), partially attributing this to constrained resources, the need to demonstrate value for money, ensuring fitness for purpose and increasing emphasis upon accountability, alongside organisational complexity. Quality is generally accepted as having two inter-related components: that of quality assurance and quality enhancement. Quality assurance is seen as being a deliberate process to review and make judgements about attainment of a quality or a given standard, thus affirming compliance. Quality enhancement can be regarded as a purposeful process of enquiry and a change or innovation leading to improvement. There is some dispute about the relationship between the two components, as highlighted in the joint enquiry in the United Kingdom (UK) by the Higher Education Academy (HEA) and the Quality Assurance Agency (QAA), within which two views predominated (HEA, 2008). The first concerned hierarchy, while in the second the concepts are separate, parallel yet mutually reinforcing, with separation based upon different drivers and funding. In the second model, quality enhancement is aligned to development of the student experience through learning and teaching innovation supported by dedicated funding and support structures (e.g. the HEA), whilst quality assurance aligns to activities undertaken as part of the HE Institution's (HEI's) own governance, supported by processes, such as the QAA. Quality assurance is viewed as more amenable to simple yes/no judgements, whilst quality enhancement requires more complex judgement.

- Quality considerations are central to all we do.
- Quality can be informed by standards.
- There is a need to determine carefully how we evidence quality assurance and enhancement.

DISCUSSION

In this discussion quality assurance and quality enhancement are regarded as part of the same concept, albeit forming a spectrum. The challenge is less about gaining consent that quality is important, than determining the purpose and effective approaches to quality assurance and enhancement. The purposes of quality are diverse, and include many elements (as demonstrated in Figure 28.1). These include securing public protection, ensuring equity, enhancing performance and sharing good practice. Quality assurance and enhancement can be seen as having a moral, economic, organisational change or transformational rationale.

Similarly, quality drivers are various, changing over time and contexts. Drivers highlighted in the literature (for example, HEA, 2008; Jackson, 2002) include:

- a competitive market, where quality can attract funding and students and enhance an organisation's reputations over a competitor's.
- funding constraints, necessitating better use of resources.
- policy changes and increased centralisation of quality control within health and education.
- changes in health professional regulations.
- demand for information to inform choice and provider selection.
- improvement of employment and economic sustainability, together with participation and inclusion policy agendas.

We cannot consider all concepts linked to quality here, but two key elements, standards and evaluation, are addressed below.

Standards

Pivotal to quality assurance is the notion of a standard against which the quality is judged. One could argue that standards are necessary because human performance tends naturally to decline or entropy over time.

The Oxford English Dictionary (2009) defines standards in a number of ways. They are seen as required, or agreed, levels of quality or attainment and as measures serving as a basis or principle to which others conform, or should conform, or by which the quality of others is judged.

Elements having particular relevance are the following. For a standard to be effective or relevant, it requires agreement or acceptance by the target community or society.

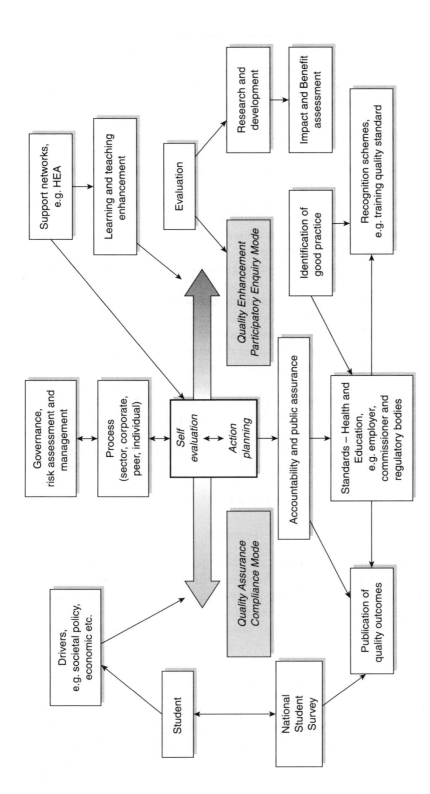

Figure 28.1 The quality map

Standards inform judgement and measurement relating to professional registration or accreditation may establish a baseline or an aspirational level of attainment and are context-specific, changing over time.

There are vast numbers of healthcare education standards. These can be classified as standards focused upon:

- an institution – the HEI's structures and/or governance arrangements which subsequently influence operational management; this includes standards acting as a reference point to inform national or sector-specific recognition or 'grading' schemes.
- an award/qualification – the required level of attainment, ensuring national/cross-institutional compatibility.
- an individual – indicating the achievement required for role recognition or entry to a professional register.
- a learning environment – identifying elements supporting effective learning.

An organisation may establish standards against one or more of the above. For example, in the UK, the QAA determines standards related to the institution, the award and the learning environment. In healthcare, it is important that standards are specific and relevant to the sector and workforce needs.

There are three other significant dimensions relating to standards. Firstly, the extent to which the standards seek to achieve consensus, for example, locally, or across nations in determining a European/International Standard, has to be considered. Secondly, there has to be appreciation of whether standards are informal, offering guidance only, or are formalised, indicating specific requirements and an agreed code of practice. Thirdly, the extent to which quality standards are complementary to, or compete with, cost reduction drives, through determining and changing controllable variables, has to be a factor in assuring and enhancing quality.

Evaluation

For robust quality approaches a systematic, evidence-based approach and evaluative thinking is required, making the link to evaluation inevitable. Jackson (2002) suggests that evaluation processes can support quality enhancement. These include: compliance audit; periodic review; annual programme review; good practice; satisfaction surveys; benchmarking; peer observation and self evaluation.

Control – who's in the driving seat?

Asking for whom quality is undertaken, or who is in control, is complex. One or more stakeholders may claim this position at any one time. Stakeholders (including the public, students and education commissioners) can turn to a range of external indicators or reference points for different aspects of quality. In HE, generally, the institution itself is accepted as being in primary control, responsible for its own standards, enforced through its own governance structures – leading in latter years to a greater focus upon quality enhancement (Jackson, 2008). The QAA is seen as having a sector-wide quality role, through the consensus of education institutions and an interface with European quality standards. Educators are also responsible, as professionals, for their own standards, or those shared by the professional community through such activity as peer review.

Equally, students can claim to be placed in the 'driving seat' as immediate learning consumers. Over recent years, the student voice has had a greater influence through involvement in institutional governance arrangements and through mechanisms such as national student surveys.

In the UK, the National Health Service (NHS) healthcare education quality is also driven by education commissioning and contractual arrangements, where particular attention is given to quality and delivery partnerships. Pittilo and Hutchinson (2001) highlighted the fact that without doubt the NHS has aimed to use quality positively as a means of achieving enhancement. Health regulators, and perhaps to a lesser extent professional bodies, also control many aspects of quality, not least the standards required for entry and continuation on professional registers, informed by public and professional consultation.

Dependent upon who is in control, failure to meet standards can result in various sanctions, with different implications for the institution, resulting perhaps in a loss of funding, reputation, market share or removal of the right to provide services.

Evidencing quality

Central to quality assurance and enhancement is the need to evidence quality claims to others. The following offers some guidance:

- use existing, accessible, current and relevant evidence, cross-referenced to relevant claims/standards.
- include all stakeholder/partners perspectives (including students and employers).
- evidence both outcomes and process (qualitative and quantitative sources).
- avoid the presentation of extra and unnecessary evidence.
- evidence good practice, sustainability, partnership working as well as actions addressing where standards are not met.
- demonstrate alignment to relevant policies, and governance, including confidentiality and data protection requirement.

CASE STUDY

Various stakeholders are involved in a quality review of post-qualifying programmes at a local HEI. The chair of the review panel assigns various responsibilities, including the following.

Mark Chopra, the student representative, concentrates on the student experience. His questions to the programme management team include the following:

- Can I access reliable, and nationally comparable, information about the quality of this university?
- Are the teaching and resources up to date?
- How can I be sure the assessments I have to do are relevant and fair?
- What particular support can I expect around my personal needs?
- How will my views about the course be listened to and acted on?
- What do current students say about the quality of the course?

The practice representative, Tanzim Williams, asks about the following elements:

- How are my specific needs met, offering relevant courses in a flexible way according to my stipulated standards?
- What is the evidence of capacity, capability and sustainability?
- Am I getting value for money?
- Is there good governance and a willingness to learn from employer/learner views?
- How will this provision enhance my services in the required way?
- Are there clear communication and liaison arrangements?
- Are robust and accessible Accreditation of Prior Learning processes in place?
- Are there clear arrangements to support equality and diversity?

The HEI's Quality and Academic Standards representative, Beverly Kirtain, raises the following:

- Are the university's quality and governance policies/arrangements clearly being applied, including joint ownership in the case of work-based learning?
- Have risks been assessed and managed?
- Have required external/internal standards been met?
- Are written action plans in place to address issues arising from evaluation?
- How will progress against the agreed action plans be monitored?
- What arrangements are in place to recognise and address non-achievement against the agreed action plans?
- What issues have been identified through evaluation that will need consideration in future plans to enhance provision and future capabilities?
- How is good practice recognised and disseminated?

CONCLUSION

The healthcare education quality landscape is complex and changing. Quality is as much about culture and values as it is about process and formal standards.

As affirmed by Clare Chapman, the NHS Director General of Workforce, 'You can't squeeze high-quality care out of a low-quality workplace' (Chapman, 2009: 20).

Healthcare education has to be responsive to the culture and quality demands of both education and health sectors addressing wide-ranging needs and skill requirements. Achievement of quality is dependent upon informed education staff, personally committed to quality.

> the quality job he didn't think anyone was going to see, is seen and the person who sees it feels a little better because of it, and is likely to pass that feeling on to others, and in that way the quality tends to keep on going. (Pirsig, 1999: 357)

See also: assessment; curriculum planning and development; feedback and marking; learning environments; management of modules and programmes; professional accountability

FURTHER READING

Fry, H., Ketteridge, S. and Marshall, S. (eds) (2009) *A Handbook for Teaching and Learning in Higher Education: Enhancing Academic Practice*. London: Taylor and Francis.

REFERENCES

Chapman, C. (2009) 'A healthy constitution', *People Management Magazine*, 29 (January): 20.

Jackson, B. (2008) 'Quality Assurance and quality enhancement – relationships and perspectives'. *Presentation at The Higher Education Academy/QAA/Hefce Conference*, 11th June 2008, East Midlands Conference Centre, Nottingham.

Jackson, N. (2002) *Updating Enhancement*. University of Surrey: Learning and Teaching Support Network.

Higher Education Academy (2008) *Quality Enhancement and Assurance – A Changing Picture?* London: QAA and the Higher Education Academy Joint Working Group.

Oxford English Dictionary (2009) Retrieved from OED website: www.askoxford.com

Pirsig, R. (1999) *Zen and the Art of Motorcycle Maintenance*, 25th anniversary edn. London: Vintage.

Pittilo, R.M. and Hutchinson, L. (2001) *The Enhancement of Quality in Higher Education – Implications for Healthcare Education and Training*. University of Surrey: Learning and Teaching Support Network.

Stoddart, J. (2004) 'Foreword', in R. Brown (ed.), *Quality Assurance in Higher Education: The UK Experience since 1992*. London: Routledge Falmer. pp. x–xiii.

Sue Lillyman

DEFINITION

Reflection and reflective practice are not new concepts to healthcare and education but have been used, discussed and written about for the past few decades. These are complex concepts that are difficult to put into a single definition, partly owing to the differing professional disciplines including their own nuances. Johns (1995) sums up reflection when he notes that it enables practitioners to assess, understand and learn through their experiences, and Burton (2000) suggests that it formalises informal learning and development through practice. Even though definitions continue to evolve, ultimately it is the interrelation between theory and practice that is fundamental.

KEY POINTS

- Reflection is a strategy that helps the practitioner to bring theory to practice.
- A reflective practitioner is a person who constantly moves and changes practice.
- Reflective learning involves actively thinking about and learning from experience.
- Critical analysis is fundamental to reflection.
- Models of reflection are tools that provide a framework.

DISCUSSION

As people engage in educational and training programmes they are often required to use reflection as a base of learning. Although reflection has gained acceptance over time, this has not been matched by an increase in its understanding, according to Thompson and Thompson (2008). If well used, reflection can make a positive contribution to continuing professional development and professional practice (Johns and Freshwater, 2005). However, when not used well it can have a negative and even dangerous effect on practice, according to Thompson and Thompson (2008).

Reflection stems from the work of the educationalists John Dewey in the 1930s and Donald Schon in the 1980s. Dewey (1933) developed his concept of reflection through experiential learning theories by seeing inside or behind experiences or using a different viewpoint. Schon (1987) draws on the scientific knowledge and part social science of practice to bring theory and practice together, introducing the term 'professional artistry'. He suggested that reflection can bridge the gap between formal education, which he calls the 'high ground', and the complex questions and actual demands of clinical practice or 'swampy lowlands' by using reflection-in-action and reflection-on-action. He also notes that it is a way of accessing deeply embedded personal knowledge. Reflection therefore places theory and practice on an equal billing and with a two-way relationship between knowing and doing resulting in the 'knowledgeable doer'.

Reflection is not limited to education and training but also helps professional practitioners to continue to integrate theory and practice in their workplace, throughout their careers, if they are willing to learn from experience and are open-minded to change.

Critical reflection

Some authors make the distinction between reflection and 'critical' reflection (Freshwater, 2007), where they suggest that critical reflection is not only thinking but also includes some form of interrogation. However, as Thompson and Thompson (2008) note, without a critical perspective reflection may result in poor quality or dangerous practice, therefore they suggest that reflection is implicitly critical in its nature as it includes a questioning approach.

Evidence-based practice

Recently, with the emphasis on evidence-based practice some practitioners have become confused as to the role of reflection. Its role here is to help the practitioner to integrate the research findings into practice or gain a wider knowledge base and experience, adapted to suit individual circumstances.

Models of reflection

As with the definitions, practitioners are offered a variety of models of reflection that have been developed over the years. Gibbs (1988) has often been the model of choice in healthcare education as his model is based on a problem-solving cyclical approach, which for nurses is similar to the nursing process. Gibbs (1988) included six stages in his approach. This cyclical approach is consistent with the work of earlier theorists, including Kolb (1984) and Boud et al. (1985).

Johns (1994) developed a much more structured model based on a series of cue questions that practitioners systematically work their way through. Louden (1991), on the other hand, offers a synthetic approach, whilst those using a hierarchical approach include Mezirow (1981), who introduced levels of reflection. Each model offers practitioners a framework to work through their reflections. However, each model has limitations – we may not always start our reflection with an experience, as many suggest. Rather, we might start the reflective process with a potential situation or problem, for example when we think about our first day in a new clinical environment, new job or our first clinical procedure. We may reflect by developing coping strategies drawing on relevant theories to form an action plan prior to encountering the actual situation. Another criticism has been the focus on negativity as the process is often triggered by a negative event or problem. Ghaye et al. (2008) have developed a more appreciative approach to reflection in their model of Participatory and Appreciative Action and Reflection (PAAR). Practitioners are encouraged to reflect on positive aspects of practice in order to gain an appreciation of their practice as opposed to always seeming to criticise practice. Ghaye et al. (2008) include four essential, mutually supportive processes in their model. These are:

- developing an appreciative gaze.
- reframing the experience.
- building practical wisdom.
- having the ethical and moral courage to use the new way of thinking.

According to Freshwater et al. (2008), the majority of reflective models tend to adopt a similar approach, falling into three main stages, including awareness, critical analysis and the development of new perspectives. Whichever model is chosen by the practitioner it needs to be used flexibly and dynamically if it is to have any impact on the professional's practice. To facilitate this process, Johns (1994) suggests the practitioner should be supported and supervised throughout.

Strategies

To aid the learner with reflection, as well as using a model of reflection, there are a number of strategies that can be used, such as learning journals or diaries, mind mapping, critical incident analysis and portfolios. Reflection can also be done singly or as a group activity through clinical supervision or action learning sets. Learning journals/diaries can be kept for a variety of reasons, including political, professional and personal, and keeping a journal is a way of developing skills to become more accountable (Ghaye and Lillyman, 2006). Entries can be interrogated, deconstructed and re-evaluated by the practitioner to deepen awareness and enrich skilfulness, enabling practitioners to construct robust justifications for their practice and valid arguments for improving practice. Journals encourage depth and breadth of learning, which will help to develop a responsible and accountable practitioner. Committing the reflection to paper/record can also aid the practitioner in developing skills for lifelong learning and effective clinical learning, and these are, therefore, valuable tools in education.

Critical incident analysis can be used as a tool to develop knowledge, skills and attitudes, using examples taken from daily work which are recorded and critically analysed in order to evaluate the experience. From this, they can then be used to develop new action plans, integrate knowledge or develop theory from practice. Mind mapping is a more pictorial approach and may suit different individuals. Here nodes are drawn as key concepts and links are made between the nodes making relationships (Ghaye and Lillyman, 2006). The portfolio is a collection of critical incidents and abstracts from the journal, that go together to form a collection of evidence that the practitioner can put forward in support of continual professional development to meet professional body requirements.

Pros and cons of reflection

Although reflection is usually promoted as a positive approach to learning and continuing professional development there are critics. As Lumby (1998) suggests, the process is questionable in relation to its validity, reliability and generalisation due to the lack of research into how reflection actually changes practice. Newell (1994) also suggests that reflection needs to be defined in a way that allows its effects on nurses and patient care to be tested.

One of the barriers noted by practitioners includes the lack of time, and many see reflection as a luxury they cannot afford in a busy clinical life. However, as Thompson and Thompson (2008) note, where practice and theory are two distinct and separate spheres then practitioners will prioritise. However, if the one supports the other then that practice can become more focused and effective through reflection and in the long term can actually save time for the practitioner. They suggest that the busier people are, the more reflective they need to be to prevent losing sight of what they are doing and why.

Effective reflection also requires a supportive and reflective culture within the organisation that will support and promote reflection for its practitioners. Other barriers for practitioners to reflect include anxiety and fear of the process or the negativity seen by always appearing to criticise practice. Another potential danger is to over-reflect to the point where practice is avoided.

CASE STUDY

This study illustrates the use of Ghaye et al.'s (2008) appreciative model in the classroom.

Teaching large groups of student nurses about loss and dying in their elderly care module can be emotive and depressing. Therefore, storyboarding was chosen as a teaching strategy to engage the students in a reflective approach using their experiences.

The students were asked to think of an experience in the clinical situation where they were nursing a patient at the end of life or dying stage. To prevent the session becoming emotional or negative the students were asked to focus on non-emotive situations in order to maintain an 'appreciative gaze'. The students were given space, in groups of eight, to share and discuss their experiences and to reframe those experiences with their peers. In order to build a collective wisdom, the students were then invited to complete a storyboard using one story from their group that they could all share in the larger classroom. Here the students could be creative and analytical in creating their story board.

In the final stage, the story boards were shared with the larger group and lecturers facilitated the discussion by drawing out themes and commonalities; drawing on the larger group's experience to identify the theory and learning in relation to the dying patient. The students were able to learn from each other and the lecturers and to develop their own action plans to move their practice forward when dealing with dying patients and their relatives.

CONCLUSION

Reflection is a process that all individuals can use to develop professionally and personally and maintain professional accreditation as part of their day-to-day care delivery. Educators in healthcare therefore need to be reflective in their own practice and promote the development of reflective skills in their students.

See also: complexity theory; experiential and work-based learning; peer support and observation; research and scholarly activity; teaching strategies; transformative learning

FURTHER READING

Ghaye, T. and Lillyman, S. (2000) *Reflection: Principles and Practice for Healthcare Professionals*, 2nd edn. Dinton: Quay Books.
Johns, C. (2004) *Becoming a Reflective Practitioner*, 2nd edn. Oxford: Blackwell.

REFERENCES

Boud, D., Keogh, R. and Walker, D. (1985) 'Promoting reflection in learning: a model', in D. Boud, R. Keogh and D. Walker (eds), *Reflection: Turning Experience into Learning*. New York: Kogan. pp. 18–40.
Burton, A. (2000) 'Reflection: nursing's practice and education panacea?', *Journal of Advanced Nursing*, 31 (5): 1009–17.
Dewey, J. (1933) *How We Think*. Chicago: Henrey Regney.
Freshwater, D. (2007) 'Reflective practice and clinical supervision two sides of the same coin?', in V. Bishop (ed.), *Clinical Supervision in Practice*, 2nd edn. Basingstoke: Palgrave. pp. 51–75.
Freshwater, D., Taylor. B.J. and Sherwood, G. (2008) *International Textbook of Reflective Practice in Nursing*. Oxford: Blackwell.
Ghaye, T. and Lillyman, S. (2006) *Learning Journals and Critical Incidents: Reflective Practice for Health Care Professionals*, 2nd edn. Dinton: Quay Books.
Ghaye, T., Melander-Wilkman, A., Kaisare, M., Chambers, P., Bergman, U., Kostenius, C. and Lillyman, S. (2008) 'Participatory and appreciative action and reflection (PARR) democratizing reflective practices', *Reflective Practice*, 9 (4): 361–95.
Gibbs, G. (1988) *Learning by Doing: A Guide to Teaching and Learning Methods*. Oxford: Further Education Unit, Oxford Brookes University.

Johns, C. (1994) 'Guided Reflection', in A. Palmer, S. Burns and C. Bulman (eds), *Reflective Practice in Nursing: The Growth of the Professional Practitioners*. Oxford: Blackwell Scientific. pp. 110–29.

Johns, C. (1995) 'Framing learning through reflection within Carper's fundamental ways of knowing in nursing', *Journal of Advanced Nursing*, 22 (2): 226–34.

Johns, C. and Freshwater, D. (2005) *Transforming Nursing through Reflective Practice*. London: Blackwell Scientific.

Kolb, D. (1984) *Experiential Learning: Experience as the Source of Learning and Development*. Englewood Cliffs, NJ: Prentice–Hall.

Louden, W. (1991) *Understanding Teaching*. London: Cassell.

Lumby, J. (1998) 'Transforming nursing through reflective practice', in C. Johns and D. Freshwater (eds), *Transforming Nursing through Reflective Practice*. Oxford: Blackwell Scientific. pp. 91–103.

Mezirow, J. (1981) 'A critical theory of adult learning and education', *Adult Education*, 32 (1): 3–24.

Newell, R. (1994) 'Reflection: art, science or pseudo-science', *Nurse Education Today*, 14 (2): 79–81.

Schon, D. (1987) *Educating the Reflective Practitioner*. San Francisco, CA: Jossey–Bass.

Thompson, S. and Thompson, N. (2008) *The Critically Reflective Practitioner*. Basingstoke: Palgrave Macmillan.

30 research and scholarly activity

Kay Currie, Nicola Andrew and Linda Proudfoot

DEFINITION

Concepts of research and scholarship are variously defined in different settings. Often within the Higher Education (HE) sector, 'research' is aligned with national funding allocation processes and the organisation's reputation for high-quality research publications and research grant capture; conversely 'scholarship' may be conceptualised as all other intellectual activity that brings together, or synthesises, knowledge in new ways to add to the development of the discipline or subject area. In an interesting debate, Thompson and Watson (2006) discuss wider definitions of scholarship, concluding that the *discovery* of knowledge through research, the *integration* of knowledge, the *application* of knowledge and the *sharing* of knowledge through teaching should be treated as different forms of scholarship on a par with each other. The organisational context in which educators in healthcare operate will help shape the form that research and/or scholarship takes, with local policy and priorities influencing the relative balance of the various complementary and sometimes competing domains of their role.

KEY POINTS

- Healthcare educator roles may span organisational contexts, for example, clinically based, within HE Institutions (HEIs), or a combination of joint appointments.
- In a world of competing priorities, understanding the various rationales for engaging in research and scholarship is important, particularly for those working within the HE sector.
- Engaging in research and scholarly activity involves getting started, getting support and getting published.

DISCUSSION

Rationale for engaging in research and scholarship

Contemporary educators in healthcare may work in a variety of roles and settings, ranging from the specialist practice educator working exclusively within the clinical area through to the HEI-based lecturer, with a growing diversity of emerging clinical-academic posts spanning the boundaries of both organisations. When making the decision to become academics, clinicians may not fully understand the current role expectations of a lecturer within a university. Deciding to move from a career as a practitioner to one as an academic is the start of a challenging journey, involving migration from a highly structured clinical role to one of more diverse requirements encompassing research and scholarship as well as teaching.

Initially, new lecturers may worry about de-skilling and may feel that they have gone from being an expert in their own field to becoming a novice in an alien environment. Over time, most academics realise that rather than skill downgrading, new skills are acquired as prior experience and knowledge are transferred into and applied to the educational setting (Andrew et al., 2009). For novice lecturers, it is important from the beginning to develop a rounded role profile encompassing research and scholarship as well as teaching; the balance of that activity may differ depending on organisational expectations and the focus of research is likely to be on *either* clinical subject matter *or* innovation in learning and teaching, less commonly both.

Irrespective of the location or role description, healthcare educators will be concerned with providing a robust educational experience for students with the overarching aim of enhancing the care of patients and clients. Engaging with research and scholarship is essential to maintain the quality of the student experience and can be loosely categorised as falling into the following spheres:

- evidence-based teaching.
- empirical enquiry in learning and teaching (pedagogical research).
- adding to the healthcare disciplines' body of knowledge (subject research).

Getting started

The nature of professional practice in healthcare education requires educators to maintain contemporary knowledge and credibility within their discipline-specific, as well as educational, fields of practice. The concept of evidence-based healthcare focuses on the integration of professional expertise and best evidence to inform decisions, which is immediately transferable to teaching, as educators utilise existing evidence of both subject matter and pedagogical practices to create opportunities for effective learning. Educators in healthcare therefore need to develop transferable skills to enable an evidence-based approach to teaching, which includes systematic retrieval of meaningful sources of evidence, critical evaluation of appropriate evidential sources and synthesis of evidence from the subject with evidence regarding sound pedagogical practice. In other words, for evidence-based teaching, educators must engage in scholarship related to both the discipline subject and the most appropriate teaching approach to promote student learning. These skills provide a platform for educators to extend their professional practice beyond the use of best evidence in clinical practice or teaching to generating evidence through subject-based or pedagogical research.

Pedagogical research aims to contribute to, and extend, understandings of learning and teaching through systematic and robust empirical enquiry (Cohen et al., 2007). In healthcare education such enquiry is often professionally focused, reflecting issues that blend the context of both fields of practice. Educators in healthcare may already be experienced researchers; conversely, for others, competence in research practice requires the development of a repertoire of skills which enables engagement in empirical enquiry to inform teaching at local, national and international levels. This repertoire reflects knowledge and understanding of research skills and techniques, research management, the research environment, communication and networking, personal effectiveness and career management.

Whilst all healthcare educators may engage in subject-based research to a certain degree, there is an expectation that lecturers will actively contribute to their institution's overall research agenda, with most HEIs currently striving to increase their share of competitive research grants and produce world-leading or internationally relevant research. In many countries national league tables are generated that indicate the institutions' research reputation, as assessed by a variety of external indicators. As experience as a healthcare educator is gained, a lecturer may be expected to contribute to, or indeed lead, aspects of the subject-based research, as career development or promotion criteria may be linked to being able to demonstrate high-quality research outputs via publication.

Both pedagogical and subject-based research contribute positively to the student experience. Investigation into various approaches to student learning stimulates innovation in teaching practice, bringing freshness whilst providing evaluative evidence of relative effectiveness in a range of situations. Similarly, there is strong evidence that being taught by lecturers who are active in subject-based research promotes student engagement and achievement (Jenkins et al., 2007). However, whilst healthcare educators may *use* both pedagogical and subject-based research in their teaching practice, it is likely that choices will have to be made in relation to *undertaking* research within a career pathway.

Getting support

Healthcare educators will need to apply diverse skills when taking a research or scholarship idea forward from conception, through implementation or investigation to evaluation and dissemination; a range of national and international organisations and strategies can be called upon to support this process. Similarly, most HEIs will offer a range of research development training opportunities, often linked to postgraduate training programmes or internal research institutes. To illustrate, the UK Research Councils jointly signed a Concordat in 2007, which outlines key principles and a code of practice to promote and support the career development of researchers; similar mechanisms may be available in other nations.

Increasingly, communities of practice (CoP) are viewed as a constructive way of engaging in peer support and professional development through collaboration with colleagues from both academic and clinical backgrounds. A CoP is based on a social participative way of learning as the 'community acts as a vehicle for collaboration, allowing members to enter dynamic and engaged relationships with colleagues and others' (Wenger et al., 2002: 4). In most communities, members commit to the development of practice within their area of work and expertise. These communities are often virtual (although not exclusively) and offer a flexible method for extending and sharing knowledge on a local, national and international scale (Andrew et al., 2009).

Getting published

Disseminating research and scholarship is an integral and rewarding aspect of academic activity, which commonly takes the form of conference papers or article publications. Sharing work with colleagues at conferences is a valuable way of spreading the fruits of research or scholarship; however, getting there can be daunting. Choosing an appropriate conference, which includes a consideration of factors such as what one hopes to achieve from presenting, the level of formality/informality, the size of the audience and the expected format of the presentation, is a key starting point. As in everyday teaching practice, it is often possible to gain tips from watching experienced presenters in action by attending conferences as a participant, prior to taking the plunge and submitting a paper.

Being expected to contribute to the production of articles and books can also be challenging for new healthcare educators. As a starting point in this process, the following thoughts are worth noting:

- Many books, articles and websites are available that provide helpful guidance for new authors. Look at a range of these to gain inspiration.
- Think about the purpose of your article: are you trying to disseminate information to as wide an audience of practitioners as possible or aiming for a high impact rated research journal? Choosing an appropriate target journal will depend on your overall aim.
- Once you have determined your purpose, read a broad sample of articles in potential target journals to get a feel for style and content. You are more likely to be successful if you match the approach of your article to those already published.
- Carefully read the guidance to authors given by the journal you eventually select and ensure you stick to the Editor's recommendations.
- Be persistent! If your article is rejected initially, follow the reviewer's feedback and try to resubmit, either in the same or another journal.

The benefits of a mechanism for peer review within the workplace, such as a publication group, can support the development of writing skills and promote a collaborative approach. Working with others at various levels of expertise can help to take the 'fear factor' out of the writing process and allow new healthcare educators to collaborate with more experienced authors to develop a publication profile, firstly as a minor contributor, working over time towards first author status. It is worth noting, however, that one person, usually the first author, should act as article coordinator to ensure that the finished product is aligned and reads as a 'whole piece'.

CASE STUDY

Alyson began her educational career as a specialist lecturer practitioner, working primarily within the clinical area but also linked to a university and supported by both partners to undertake a Postgraduate Certificate in Education. She was later appointed to a full-time university lecturer post where she extended her qualifications by gaining an MSc in Nursing. Working full-time opened up further opportunities and Alyson attended available seminars on scholarship in learning and teaching and joined a departmental publications group, gaining support for writing up aspects of her MSc dissertation for publication and conference presentation. Encouraged by these experiences, Alyson then joined a team of researchers on an externally funded project, accepting responsibility for an area of data collection whilst gaining further insights into the research process. Gaining confidence and with an eye to future career progression, Alyson is now developing a proposal for PhD studies and hopes to build on her interest in scholarship and research in learning and teaching.

CONCLUSION

Research and scholarship should be an integral part of the healthcare educator role, whether focusing on the discipline subject base or pedagogical initiatives. Whilst the challenges in getting started, getting support and getting published should not be underestimated, there is clear evidence to demonstrate the benefits to students from contact with educators who are actively engaged in developing and contributing to the knowledge base of both healthcare and teaching practice.

See also: academic staff development; leadership and management in academia; partnership working

FURTHER READING

A wide range of relevant resources is available at the following sites:
www.heacademy.ac.uk
http://iet.open.ac.uk/research/castl.cfm
www.hefce.ac.uk/Research/ref/
www.researchconcordat.ac.uk/

REFERENCES

Andrew, N., Ferguson, D., Wilkie, G. and Simpson, L. (2009) 'Developing professional identity in nursing academics: the role of communities of practice', *Nurse Education Today* 29 (6): 607–11, published online 27th February 2009.
Cohen, L., Manion, L. and Morrison, K. (2007) *Research Methods in Education*, 6th edn. London: Routledge.
Jenkins, A., Healey, M. and Zetter, R. (2007) *Linking Teaching and Research in Disciplines and Departments*. Retrieved from HEA website: www.heacademy.ac.uk/assets/York/documents/LinkingTeachingAndResearch_April07.pdf
Thompson, D. and Watson, R. (2006) 'Professors of nursing: What do they profess?', *Nurse Education in Practice*, 6 (3): 123–6.
Wenger, E., McDermott, R. and Snyder, W. (2002) *A Guide to Managing Knowledge. Cultivating Communities of Practice*. Boston, MA: Harvard Business School Press.

31 role model

Sandra Flynn

DEFINITION

The notion of 'role model' first emerged in research concerning the socialisation of medical students by Merton (1996), who theorised that individuals will relate to an identified group of people and aspire to the social roles they occupy. Gibson further conceptualised a role model as 'a cognitive construction based on the attributes of people in social roles that an individual perceives to be similar to him or herself to some extent and desires to increase perceived similarity by emulating those attributes' (2004: 36). Placing an individual in the category of role model is often a consequence of depicting an image that others are inspired by and consequentially try to replicate; thus role modelling is seen as the heart of character formation and this in turn can direct personal and professional growth and development. In order to justify being identified as a role model, an individual needs to portray a positive attitude and image, inspiring others through what they say and what they do; by this means they earn respect for themselves and the position they occupy.

KEY POINTS

- Role modelling can be a powerful teaching tool for the dissemination of knowledge, skills and values.
- Learning from role models occurs through observation and reflection.
- Role modelling needs to be intentional and have purpose.

DISCUSSION

Role modelling in education concerns itself more with the exposure of learners to certain attitudes, lifestyles and views rather than the conveyance of knowledge (Rose, 2004). Using educators in healthcare as role models for professional behaviour has long been identified as a means of encouraging effective learning by helping to convey the attributes associated with healthcare professionals, including personal qualities such as behaviour, attitudes and values. Recognised as a significant force in the development of sound professional characteristics, appropriate role models have been identified as an essential part of health profession education (Harris, 2004).

role model

Healthcare educators can facilitate the acquisition of clinical skills and expertise in students through role modelling, but in order to do so they must be an emissary of professionalism, knowledge and professional astuteness. These qualities should be evident in their actions and strong work ethos, reflecting this commitment through their behaviour at all times (Myrick and Yonge, 2005). There are several challenges that the role model may face, including the need to actively develop the skills associated with this concept. Role modelling is not a static skill, but one that evolves and adjusts to meet the educational and professional requirements of the individual student.

Demonstrating variations in behaviour is a human trait and can be evident in role modelling; as such it is impossible for the educator role model to be a constant example of righteousness. Here the directive for the role model should be to have an awareness that their actions, positive or negative, can have an impact on students.

Being an appropriate role model may be a difficult standard to achieve; as Joffe (2005) warns, the notion of one size fits all may not apply in every situation. It is possible for educators to influence the development and growth of their students even when exhibiting poor role modelling behaviours (Lunenberg et al., 2007).

The amount of contact time an individual student spends with a role model can help contribute to the quality of the experience; too little contact time may not be enough to leave a positive impression upon the individual learner whereas too much exposure may lead to indoctrination. Getting the balance right can be difficult to accomplish but can be attained through reflecting on performance and feedback from students.

The term 'role model' can be interlinked with the term 'mentor', although there are distinct differences between the two. The distinction was simplified by Struchen and Porta (1997), who viewed role modelling and mentorship as a complementary partnership, role modelling concerning itself with individuals discovering a positive image or identity that attracts them and mentoring equipping the individual with the skills needed to attain that image. Allen and Eby (2007) noted that the main differences in the roles related to the amount of support provided, and the bonds formed, stating that they can range in the mentor-protégé relationship from a moderate to an intense level, whereas they are non-existent in the role model-observer relationship; interaction between mentor and protégé is necessary, but is not necessary in the role model–observer relationship.

According to Gunderman (2002) good role models perform three main tasks: they exhibit behaviour that strengthens the constructive behaviour of others; their conduct helps students to resist developing destructive behaviours; and their actions help inform the practice of the student.

The concept of learning by observation was described by Bandura (1977, 1986), who suggested that role modelling assists individuals in learning new behaviours without the need for trial and error. In order for this to happen, certain conditions need to exist for individuals to learn and effectively model

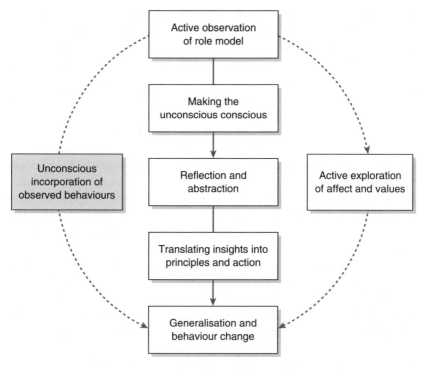

Figure 31.1 Systematic representation of the process of role modelling (Cruess et al., 2008)

behaviour; the learner needs to be attentive, be able to remember what they observed (retention), be able to replicate the behaviour (reproduction) and have a good reason to imitate the observed behaviour (motivation). This observation is perceived by the learner as new behaviour which is retained and then, at a later date, is used to inform and guide practice.

What role models do is likely to have more of an impact upon learners than what they say. Westberg and Jason (1993) state that when students observe role models engaging in behaviours and tasks that they associate with their future work, they consciously and unconsciously focus on what they do and say. This complex mix of conscious and unconscious interpretation is represented in Figure 31.1

The ability of processing the characteristics of a role model takes place via two different routes, which include an active thought process leading to change, followed by active reflection where thoughts are frequently communicated in abstract terms. As a result, an emotion can change from unconscious to conscious, effectively being converted into principles and actions.

The left-hand route of Figure 31.1 demonstrates the process of how observed behaviours are unconsciously integrated into the learner's own behaviours and ideals. Fundamental to the success and effectiveness of role modelling is the educator's appreciation of the power of the unconscious observation (Cruess et al., 2008). Competent behaviour is more likely to be imitated if a mutual relationship is established between the role model and the learner. However, it is essential for role models to be aware that they are the epitome of what students are trying to become and therefore their behaviour is open to scrutiny at all times, both in and out of the learning environment.

A student's theoretical aims and ambitions can be brought to life by a good role model; this is especially important when trying to achieve the types of delicate and complex goals that cannot be expressed in words. For example, certain aspects of behaviour such as showing empathy are difficult to explain but can be demonstrated more effectively in everyday practice (Westberg and Jason, 1993). Likewise, by sharing personal experiences, feelings and values the role model can engage learners in aspects of behaviour that cannot readily be displayed.

There are several methods through which educators can model beliefs and values to students, integrating the best of the rhetoric into their teaching in a manner whereby they are ultimately living the example. Practical demonstrations, role-play, case studies and group discussions are valuable, stimulating and memorable means of modelling practice. In these learning situations students can act out behaviours and attitudes through simulation or discussion of actual case situations allowing for appropriate responses to be debated after each scenario (Judkins and Eldridge, 2001). Cruess et al. (2008) identify the following abilities required in order to facilitate the role: clinical competence, teaching skills and personal qualities (see Table 31.1). Clinical competence includes the educator's ability to deliver reliable clinical judgement and decision making. Teaching skills are essential in the transmission of clinical competence; the approach should be student-centred, incorporating effective communication, providing feedback and facilitating reflection. Personal qualities including compassion, honesty and integrity are all attributes that promote learning. Importantly, educators should be able to promote good interpersonal relationships, have an enthusiasm for practice and teaching, and constantly strive for excellence.

CASE STUDY

Maria is a hospital-based Consultant Nurse. As part of her role she is involved with the professional and personal development of a range of staff from medical and nursing students to qualified healthcare professionals. Maria regularly works with individuals on a one-to-one basis, giving staff the opportunity to observe and discuss her practice, including her clinical expertise, interpersonal skills and professional values within the surgical specialty.

Often the staff are quite nervous in their approach to the experience and are unsure how to deal with certain problems they encounter. Maria interacts

Table 31.1 The characteristics of role modelling

Positive characteristics	Negative characteristics
Clinical competence	
Excellent knowledge and skills	Deficient knowledge and skills
Effective communication	Ineffective communication
Sound clinical reasoning	Poor clinical reasoning
Teaching skills	
Aware of role	Unaware of role
Explicit about what is modelled	Not explicit about what is modelled
Makes time for teaching	Does not make time for teaching
Shows respect for student needs	Does not show respect for student needs
Provides timely feedback	Does not provide timely feedback
Encourages reflection in students	Does not encourage reflection in students
Personal qualities	
Compassionate and caring	Insensitive to patient's suffering
Displays honesty and integrity	Lapses in honesty and integrity
Enthusiastic for own practice	Dissatisfaction with own practice
Effective interpersonal skills	Ineffective interpersonal skills
Commitment to excellence	Acceptance of mediocre results
Collegial	Lack of collegiality
Demonstrates humour	Humourless approach

Source: Cruess et al., 2008

with the individuals throughout, reflecting on practice and placing emphasis on good communication skills with each other and the patient. She encourages the learners to problem-solve and actively participate in the learning process.

Maria relates her own positive and negative experiences to the learners, which she substantiates with personal examples, discussing how she overcame each problem and what she learnt. She gives consistent and constructive feedback, both positive and negative, whilst at the same time valuing the comments and contributions of the students. At the end of their time together, she provides opportunities for the learners to reflect on and discuss their abilities and achievements and their development needs.

CONCLUSION

Role modelling should be viewed as a healthy route to development (Gibson, 2004), as it is important for educators to seize any opportunity to model the positive characteristics learners want to develop, but importantly there must be a true consistency between what is said and what is actually demonstrated. Inconsistencies can lead only to negative modelling; students need to observe and develop a clear vision of a good role model, so that they in turn will adopt similar personal and professional traits.

role model

See also: clinical competence; experiential learning; learning environments; mentorship; practice teaching; reflection

FURTHER READING

Beauchamp, T.L. and Childress, J.R. (2001) *Principles of Biomedical Ethics*, 5th edn. New York: Oxford University Press.

Rose, M. and Best, D. (2005) *Transforming Practice through Clinical Education, Professional Supervision and Mentoring*. London: Churchill Livingstone.

REFERENCES

Allen, T.D. and Eby, L.T. (2007) *The Blackwell Handbook of Mentoring: A Multiple Perspectives Approach*. Malden, MA and Oxford, UK: Blackwell.

Bandura, A. (1977) *Social Learning Theory*. London: Prentice–Hall.

Bandura, A. (1986) *Social Foundations of Thought and Action*. London: Prentice–Hall.

Cruess, S., Cruess, R. and Steinert, Y. (2008) 'Role modeling: making the most of a powerful teaching strategy', *British Medical Journal*, 336: 718–21.

Gibson, D.E. (2004) 'Role models in career development: new directions for theory and research', *Journal of Vocational Behaviour*, 65: 134–56.

Gunderman, R.B. (2002) 'Role models in the education of radiologists', *American Journal of Roentgenology* 179: 327–9. Retrieved from www.ajronline.org/cgi/content/full/179/2/327

Harris, G.D. (2004) 'Professionalism: Part 1 – Introduction and being a role model', *Family Medicine*, 36 (5): 314–15.

Joffe, B. (2005) 'Models of clinical education', in M. Rose and D. Best, *Transforming Practice through Clinical Education, Professional Supervision and Mentoring*. London: Elsevier Health Sciences. pp. 29–37.

Judkins, S.K. and Eldridge, C. (2001) 'Let's put "caring" back into healthcare: teaching staff to care', *Journal of Nursing Administration*, 31 (11): 509–11.

Lunenberg, M., Korthagen, F. and Swennen, A. (2007) 'The teacher educator as a role model', *Teaching and Teacher Education*, 23: 586–601.

Merton, R. (1996) *On Social Structure and Science*. New York: University of Chicago Press.

Myrick, F. and Yonge, O. (2005) *Nursing Preceptorship: Connecting Practice and Education*. Philadelphia, PA: Lippincott, Williams and Wilkins.

Rose, D. (2004) *The Potential of Role-model Education: The Encyclopedia of Informal Education*. Retrieved from www.infed.org/biblio/role_model education.htm

Struchen, W. and Porta, M. (1997) 'From role-modeling to mentoring for African American youth: ingredients for successful relationships', *Preventing School Failure*, 41: 119–23.

Westberg, J. and Jason, H. (1993) *Collaborative Clinical Education: The Foundation of Effective Health Care*. London: Springer.

key concepts in healthcare education

32 service user and carer involvement

Terry Williams and Dianne Phipps

DEFINITION

User and/or carer involvement in Higher Education (HE) can mean different things to different people, usually concerning the way that users/carers of human services are involved in education, and in the amount of that involvement.

Users/carers are an integral part of the learning experience for students studying healthcare because, ultimately, they are the people with whom the qualifying students are going to interact on a daily basis during their professional career. It is true also that, for people who identify themselves as professionals, they too will be users of services and often carers too. So why involve people who are identified as users/carers within HE? The answer lies somewhat in the notion that users/carers often do not have the same insight into the political and procedural world of public services as those who work within their structures on a day-to-day basis, but what they do have, and this is why their input is invaluable, is knowledge of what it is like to be on the receiving end of human services. This knowledge can be utilised in various ways during students' HE journey, so that when they are ultimately working in the 'real' world, the user and carer voice will be the one sought and listened to during episodes of care or support, and the nature of those episodes of care or support will aim to be very much that of a partnership.

KEY POINTS

- Involvement of users and carer of human services within HE is evolving and, while challenging, can have real benefits for all involved.
- Partnership working between users/carers and HE institutions involves practical issues that can enhance the process and need careful attention to ensure partnership working is as successful as possible.

DISCUSSION

This discussion has been written using both HE and user/carer representation. It therefore contains both empirical evidence and personal accounts.

The involvement of users/carers in human services can be traced back to the early 19th century (Rush, 2004), when ex-patients were employed to care for and advise on the treatment of patients receiving interventions. The following decades brought major changes in both social and health policy, with the user becoming the receiver of services, often having little or no say in the delivery or development of interventions. Some users began to question this situation, lobbying for a greater say in their treatment or support. User/carer involvement in HE can be seen to parallel attempts at full citizen participation within a democracy, engaging and including people throughout, whilst trying to reduce the degree of tokenism experienced (Arnstein, 1969).

Within HE Institutions (HEIs), this ethos of participation has gained momentum and support within recent years. Some of this support relates to the benefits reported by students who have experienced the inclusion of users/carers within a programme of education; benefits such as having the time and facilitative environment to examine issues from the user/carer's perspective which in turn may have an impact upon the attitudes of students, with consideration of empowering users/carers to be active in their own health or support needs (Happell and Roper, 2003).

Whilst the benefits of involving users/carers in HE are beginning to be recognised, the process does not always happen without barriers to working in partnership, and with effort needed to ensure that the involvement is real and not tokenistic (Lathlean et al., 2006). HEIs should endeavour to develop a genuine partnership with service users and carers based upon equality. Participation should be an empowering experience for all parties. This participation is enhanced by having in place not only 'champions' for the cause of users/carers involvement, but also knowledge of underlying principles for partnership working and some thought given to the practicalities of involvement.

Working in Partnership: issues for consideration

An example of a successful partnership arrangement between users, carers and HE is that of the Forum of Carers and Users of Services (FOCUS), which works with universities throughout the Cheshire and Merseyside area in the United Kingdom, providing valuable advice and support to health and social care programmes of education.

In a consultation carried out by FOCUS, it was highlighted that particular importance was given to good communication with lecturers and other HE staff, provision of appropriate support and having opportunities for training and development. Most of the issues raised were similar to those contained in the document 'The Eight Principles' (Commission for Social Care Inspection (CSCI), 2007). The General Social Care Council, Skills for Care and the Social Care Institute for Excellence regard these eight principles which, while pertaining to social care have equal relevance to healthcare, as the minimum standards for involving service users and carers in their work. These are as follows (CSCI, 2007):

- We will be clear about the purpose of involving service users or carers in aspects of our work.
- We will work with people who use social care and health services to agree the way they are involved.
- We will let service users and carers choose the way they become involved.
- We will exchange feedback about the outcome of service users' and carers' involvement in appropriate ways.
- We will try to recognise and overcome barriers to involvement.
- We will make every effort to include the widest possible range of people in our work.
- We will value the contribution, expertise and time of service users and carers.
- We will use what we have learnt from working with service users and carers to influence changes in our ways of working, to achieve better outcomes.

In practice, this means that good informal communication is vital, particularly clarity regarding what is expected of the service user/carer and the expected learning outcomes of teaching sessions. Carers and service users expect to be well informed as this reduces anxiety and promotes working in a genuine partnership. They need to know details regarding times, rooms, car parking and who will meet them when they arrive. Consideration should be given to providing refreshments. Where the communication is informal, it is easier for the carer or service user to raise issues of concern or simply ask for more information, such as maps of the campus.

Honesty and openness is considered important, so that service users and carers are able to express concerns, differences and problems in an open way. Individual needs should be considered; for example, some service users may have a condition that means that they need to take regular refreshments. Wheelchair users will need to park near the venue and where necessary someone will need to escort them from their car. Effective communication on arrival is necessary so that the service user is not kept waiting.

Support and feedback are very important. For many people, speaking before a group of students or speaking out at a meeting takes a certain amount of courage. Support should be available before and after each session. Also, it is important that carers and service users receive feedback and acknowledgement. They often need reassurance that their contribution was valued but they also want feedback so that they can become more effective and/or strive to improve their next presentation. Valuing people involves treating them with respect and paying appropriate fees. Normally the visiting lecturer rate is applicable.

Range of Participation

The most common method of involvement is teaching, but many service users and carers are interested in participating in other activities. They can contribute to planning and evaluating modules and programmes or participate in interviewing course applicants. They can also attend Boards of Studies and take part in programme development and validations. As with all areas of involvement the basic principles outlined above should be applied and the HEI should facilitate participation. Developing a participative culture and making adjustments in methods of communication and in power relationships are desirable to ensure that participation is meaningful.

In using service users and carers to teach students, it can be valuable for them to tell their story. This usually includes information on their illness or condition, the effect on their lives and how they cope with the associated problems. Often they will talk about why they needed services, what services they received, what was helpful, what other help they felt they should have had, whether the professionals involved were supportive and whether they communicated effectively.

Service users and carers can also be used more imaginatively. Students, working in small groups, can be given a task such as undertaking an assessment on a service user. The service user can then give feedback on the quality of communication and other issues. For some programmes, comments on the quality and relevance of the assessment can help the students to improve their skills. Another example is where the carer or service user observes students discussing a case study, and then gives a carer or service user perspective.

Whatever approach is used, the involvement of service users and carers has a significant influence on students. Involvement develops a deeper understanding of service users' and carers' needs and perceptions. In particular, it brings a greater sense of realism.

CASE STUDY

Leslie is planning a new programme, and is very much aware of the benefits of involving users/carers within the HE environment. Leslie carefully plans the modules to include sessions with user/carer involvement and is commended for this at the validation event. Following validation, Leslie liaises with a group of user/carer representatives, with whom he has a good relationship, and talks to them about the new modules within the validated programmes, pointing out where he has included particular sessions that could be user/carer led. The user/carer group think that the programme looks good, and work with Leslie on collating content for the module. They do say, however, that next time they should be involved with the programme from the beginning, as they have some ideas that will be difficult to include as the validated content is now set.

On reflection, Leslie realises that he excluded the user/carer group at the outset, a thing which he was always keen not to do. When Leslie examined why he had done so, he was surprised to realise that it was because he thought that this part of the process was an academic's role, and that he had mirrored in his actions some of the uneven power relationships between user/carer and professionals in practice that he always tried to avoid.

CONCLUSION

User and carer involvement is developing within each HEI at different paces and with differing support or drivers. For user/carer involvement to become a clear partnership, those involved should be mindful not only of 'The Eight Principles' (CSCI, 2007), but also of the need to listen to users and carers and to work with them to ensure systems are in place to support the involvement running smoothly. Benefits to user/carer involvement will outweigh any barriers, and the involvement will be meaningful and have a real impact, not only upon the students, but upon their future work as professionals, the organisations and cultures in which they work, their colleagues, the multi-disciplinary team, and ultimately, each and every one of us.

See also: clinical competence; curriculum planning and development; management of modules and programmes; partnership working

FURTHER READING

McPhail, M. (ed.) (2008) *Service User and Carer Involvement: Beyond Good Intentions.* Edinburgh: Dunedin Academic Press.

REFERENCES

Arnstein, S. (1969) 'A ladder of citizen participation', *Journal of the American Institute of Planners*, 35: 216–24.

CSCI (2007) 'Eight Principles to Involvement'. Retrieved from CSCI website: www.ncvo-vol. org.uk/campaigningeffectiveness/projects/index.asp?id=10494

Happell, B. and Roper, C. (2003) 'The role of a mental health consumer in the education of postgraduate psychiatric nursing students: the students' evaluation', *Journal of Psychiatric and Mental Health Nursing*, 10 (3): 343–50.

Lathlean, J., Burgess, A., Coldham, T., Gibson, C., Herbert, L., Levett-Jones, T., Simons, L. and Tee, S. (2006) 'Experiences of service user and carer participation in healthcare education', *Nurse Education Today*, 26: 732–7.

Rush, B. (2004) 'Mental health service user involvement in England: lessons from history', *Journal of Psychiatric and Mental Health Nursing*, 11: 313–18.

service user and carer involvement

33 simulated learning and objective structured clinical examinations

Andrea McLaughlin

DEFINITION

Simulated learning is learning that occurs in an environment which is as close to the 'real life' situation as possible, providing students with opportunities for the development of professional skills and helping them to increase their confidence in delivering high-quality care. Simulation usually occurs within well-equipped skills laboratories. Skills may be practised using models and simulators, or in some cases, by students, staff and actors engaging in role-play. Simulated learning is a major part of many healthcare programmes and, in addition to aiding skills development, there is opportunity to use it for assessment of students by formulating Objective Structured Clinical Examinations (OSCEs) which are skills-based.

OSCEs have been used to assess medical students for more than 30 years (Rushforth, 2007), and are increasingly included within programmes of education for other health professionals. The OSCE is an examination that focuses on a practical task or problem, where students are expected to demonstrate their practical skills and competence, often within a given time frame. Many healthcare programmes contain practice elements and the OSCE is a useful tool in assessing the acquisition of skills and clinical competence in practice, although evidence suggests that OSCEs are traditionally completed under simulated conditions such as skills laboratories (Green and Cook, 2005; Rushforth, 2007).

KEY POINTS

- Simulation must mirror the 'real' situation as closely as possible.
- Objectives must be measurable and achievable.
- Clinical focus and application to practice must be evident throughout.
- Examination must include formative and/or summative assessment of students' performance.

DISCUSSION

Simulated learning can take a variety of forms, such as observing and then copying a skill, participation in skills workshops, 'skills drills' or dealing with a given scenario. The emphasis for the teacher should be that students must be able to justify their actions and not merely learn how to perform the skill (Jay, 2007; Khattab and Rawlings, 2001). Important too is that all equipment used within simulations should be of good quality, well maintained and be up to date (Jay, 2007). When OSCEs are used, the assessment tool is developed by formulating the OSCE, which, as the name suggests, is structured around objectives the student has to meet. The OSCE documentation must be clearly and logically set out, so the student is aware of the order in which to perform the steps of the OSCE, and exactly what has to be achieved. This also serves as an *aide-memoire* for the student and assessor. Each statement should be measurable, thus informing the student and the assessor of the acceptable standard that must be attained, thus avoiding ambiguity. A system for marking the OSCE must be decided upon, as there are a number of approaches from which to choose (Rushforth, 2007). Traditionally, OSCEs take place within a skills laboratory, with each student undertaking the same task or group of tasks, with assessment by the same group of assessors. The assessment has to be completed within a given time limit (Khattab and Rawlings, 2001), and may be formative or summative. The skills assessed may be single skills, such as hand washing, or multiple skills. OSCE assessment may comprise a series of work-stations within a teaching facility, for example a skills laboratory or a clinic.

Assessment can occur throughout a module or programme, at a progression point or at the end. OSCEs can be introduced early in a programme to allow the student to move from the simple to the complex, to increase their confidence and competence and to link theory with practice (Green and Cook, 2005).

Assessment of OSCEs usually involves lecturers, but should also include practitioners; working in partnership is a sound approach, with assessment teams of lecturers and practice staff working together (Green and Cook, 2005; Jay, 2007).

Assessors need to be appropriately prepared and developed so they are confident and objective in the assessment process. Standardised mentor/ assessor preparation can be difficult to achieve (Green and Cook, 2005) but is paramount to eliminate problems. Some assessors may find it difficult to fail students or give low marks (Duffy, 2004; Green and Cook, 2005), but adequate preparation and support may help to resolve this.

Benefits

Simulated learning can be beneficial for teaching skills that are difficult to achieve in practice but are mandatory for the student, if the 'real' situation is not appropriate or available. Examples include competence in resuscitation where students simulate the skill using models. Students have reported that simulated learning develops their critical thinking skills and application of knowledge to practice (Leung et al., 2008). This is congruent with theories relating to skills acquisition, which propose that students learn theory first, often in a classroom setting, progressing to demonstration of the skill in a controlled environment such as a skills laboratory. The students then acquire the skill through practice, again within the controlled environment, and subsequently observe, simulate and practise the skill in the practice area. This also takes account of any idiosyncrasies that may exist in the practice area and the fact that procedures in practice may differ slightly from one practice area to another.

One advantage of OSCEs is that, in theory, all students undertake the same assessment. The marking sheet for an OSCE provides a checklist for both student and assessor, so the skill can be practised prior to summative assessment, and students are aware of exactly what is expected of them (Khattab and Rawlings, 2001). When used within a skills laboratory setting, the fact that the OSCE is carried out using the same equipment and is normally assessed by the same assessors facilitates objectivity in the assessment process (Jay, 2007; Khattab and Rawlings, 2001). Although OSCEs are traditionally used to assess clinical skills, professional issues such as the evidence base for practice, accountability or ethical considerations can be built in to the OSCE. This is advantageous in that the student's knowledge of research and ethics can be considered for every skill, thus integrating these subjects into the programme and fostering the application of theory into practice. Additionally, students may be expected to communicate with the assessor during the OSCE and provide a justification for their actions (Guillaume, 2003; Jay, 2007; Khattab and Rawlings, 2001). OSCEs can increase the student's ability to learn actively and students have reported that OSCE assessment is positive as it shows their abilities (Green and Cook, 2005).

Challenges and limitations

Simulated learning has been criticised for being unrealistic, particularly when the 'client' is a piece of equipment (Jay, 2007). Thus, the environment should be as realistic as possible, and students should dress as they would in the practice area; however, scepticism and inability to make the transition from simulation to reality has been reported (Baxter et al., 2009). Challenges for OSCEs include marking, which has been widely discussed and debated (Rushforth, 2007), with many opting for simple criteria such as 'pass/fail', or a more detailed marking system that includes numerical scoring. Either way, a decision has to be made regarding the pass mark, or whether certain steps of the OSCE must be passed, or, as is the case in some OSCEs, whether a mark of 100% is needed for a pass. This can be problematic as assigning a full range of marks to every OSCE would be impracticable. Assessment should always be as easy as possible to administer, therefore for practical purposes

OSCEs may be marked as 'pass' or 'fail'. Whatever the decision, the proviso that unsafe practice will equate to an automatic fail may be included.

The issue of whether OSCEs within simulated situations actually mirror what occurs in practice has been raised (Freeth and Fry, 2005; Green and Cook, 2005). Duffy (2004) pointed out that assessment should capture the quality of the students' performance. The answer, maybe, is to have OSCEs assessed in practice areas, as practice skills should be tested rigorously (Green and Cook, 2005) and assessment in contrived simulated settings may not give a true assessment of a student's performance. This is supported by Brennan and Hutt, who state that 'nurses in practice need to regain control of nurse education' (2001: 187). This, however, is not an easy solution, as any assessment has to be standardised, easy to use and with the consideration that elimination of bias may be problematic.

Assessment in practice

The OSCE is an ideal method for assessing skills in practice, although it has its advantages and disadvantages. As an OSCE is essentially a measure of performance in practice, it can be argued that it should take place in the practice setting and student performance should be judged by appropriately trained practice assessors, working together with educators where possible. Overall though, the student has to demonstrate the ability to manage complex situations in practice, albeit with support.

The OSCE is a detailed assessment that confirms a student's competence in a given skill. OSCEs may link to, and be derived from, the standards required by the various professional bodies that govern healthcare staff, and as such may provide the foundation for grading practice. Rushforth stated that it is often the case that 'excellent performance cannot enhance a student's final grade' (2007: 486), but innovative use of OSCE within the practice setting could change this, so that all aspects of student performance are reflected in the final mark or degree classification.

CASE STUDY

A cohort of student nurses needs to demonstrate skills relating to ward management. It is logical to assess the students' managerial skills within the practice setting as this does not lend itself to simulation in a skills lab. An OSCE was developed, in a partnership of academic and clinical staff, which included: students allocating workloads to staff; organising workload for part of a shift; liaising with medics and other health professionals; conducting a ward round; administration of medicine; record keeping and documentation. A detailed marking schedule was developed to guide the assessors and provide feedback for the students.

For the OSCE the students took charge of their placements with the mentor working alongside as an assessor; a second assessor was also present. The academic link lecturers attended after the OSCE process was complete to discuss the students' progress with the assessors and the students, and to act as moderators. In addition, the external examiner was given the opportunity to attend a sample of the OSCEs to confirm the quality of the assessment process.

CONCLUSION

Simulated learning is a valuable tool for promoting skills acquisition. It facilitates the development of practice and enables students to become familiar with procedures and equipment within a safe environment, prior to working in the practice area.

Efforts must be made to make the experience positive and as realistic as possible, and both academic and practice-based staff should contribute to the assessment of students. Once skills have been assimilated, then OSCE can be employed either within the skills laboratory or the practice area, to ascertain students' competence. Marking and assigning grades to OSCE assessment remains a source of debate.

See also: assessment; clinical competence; experiential and work-based learning; teaching strategies

FURTHER READING

Rushforth, H. (2007) 'Objective structured clinical examination: review of literature and implications for nursing education', *Nurse Education Today*, 27 (5): 481–90.

REFERENCES

Baxter, P., Akhtar-Danesh, N., Valaitis, R., Stanyou, W. and Sproul, S. (2009) 'Simulated experiences: nursing students share their perspectives', *Nurse Education Today*, 29 (8): 859–66. Retrieved from www.sciencedirect.com/science

Brennan, A.M. and Hutt, R. (2001) 'The challenges and conflicts of facilitating learning in practice: the experiences of two clinical nurse educators', *Nurse Education in Practice*, 1 (4): 181–8.

Duffy, K. (2004) *Failing Students.* London: NMC.

Freeth, D. and Fry, H. (2005) 'Nursing students' and tutors' perceptions of teaching in a clinical skills centre', *Nurse Education Today*, 25 (4): 272–82.

Green, S. and Cook, D. (2005) 'Examining skills and practice', *Midwives*, 9: 478–80.

Guillaume, A. (2003) 'Nursing students and lecturers perspectives of objective structured clinical examination', *Nurse Education Today*, 23 (6): 419–26.

Jay, A. (2007) 'Students perception of the OSCE: a valid assessment tool?' *British Journal of Midwifery*, 15: 32–7.

Khattab, A.D. and Rawlings, B. (2001) 'Assessing nurse practitioner students using a modified objective structured clinical examination', *Nurse Education Today*, 21 (7): 541–50.

Leung, S.F., Mok, E. and Wong, D. (2008) 'The impact of assessment methods on the learning of students', *Nurse Education Today*, 28 (6): 711–19.

Rushforth, H. (2007) 'Objective structured clinical examination: review of literature and implications for nursing education', *Nurse Education Today*, 27 (5): 481–90.

Bernadette Gartside

DEFINITION

Whilst research, theories and opinions inevitably vary regarding the concept of dyslexia, there is universal agreement that developmental dyslexia has both a genetic and neurological base, and furthermore, that language processing and working memory difficulties result in noticeable problems with literacy unconnected to general or intellectual capability. The Department for Education and Skills (DfES) (2005) emphasises typical characteristics associated with dyslexia, including the disparity of skills inherent within an individual that influences the manner and speed with which information is received, stored, retrieved and ultimately formed. Certainly, the importance of considering the strengths and weaknesses of an individual are vital, not only in terms of the learning process but also when considering the often hidden, yet fundamentally entwined, emotional and psychological aspects.

KEY POINTS

- Access to assessment and early intervention is key to developing strategies to support individual learning needs.
- Disclosure and perceived implications, both within academia and professional practice, are a genuine concern for many students with Specific Learning Difficulties (SpLD).
- Obstacles in the way information is processed inhibit the ability to assimilate information promptly and efficiently.
- Metacognitive awareness is a fundamental characteristic within the learning process.

DISCUSSION

When entering Higher Education many individuals are unaware that the difficulties they experience may be associated with a SpLD such as dyslexia. Nor indeed are they fully aware of the challenges that this may pose (Richardson and Wydell, 2003), both in an academic and working environment. Reid and Kirk (2001) recognise the importance of metacognition within the learning process, stating this can lead to increased confidence, and promote autonomy alongside ability.

White (2007) cautions against viewing the issues surrounding dyslexia as solely related to academia, stressing the importance of transferring skills into the workplace, including the provision of tailored support in practice to meet individual specific needs. Under the Disability Discrimination Act (Office of Public Sector Information, 2005) and the Disability Equality Duty (Office for Disability Issues, 2006), responsible bodies are required by law to make reasonable adjustments to ensure that a disabled student is not placed at a substantial disadvantage. Universities must anticipate what sort of adjustments may be necessary for a disabled student in the future and, where appropriate, make adjustments in advance, including placement provision.

Assessment and support framework

Early assessment and intervention adopting a holistic perspective is essential to obtain recognition of need. However, although an individual is well aware of the difficulties he or she is experiencing, the reality of the process of identification and being seen as 'disabled' can raise issues of self esteem, competence, stigma and so forth (Jamieson and Morgan, 2008; Tinklin et al., 2002), highlighting that individual needs are not solely restricted to cognitive or literacy difficulties. To ensure clarity it is important to highlight the difference between the screening process (gathers information and evidence), as opposed to diagnostic assessment (analytically identifies the difficulties and suggests recommendations).

The Assessment Framework (Table 34.1) is a typical representation of the process within the United Kingdom, from referral through to identification and subsequent teaching and learning; illustrating not only procedure and possible intervention, but also highlighting emotional and psychological aspects.

The process of assessment is complex and involves a range of individuals, including educational psychologists, diagnostic assessors, specialist teachers and disability officers. It is important to note that each stage of this process may be carried out by any of the above, depending upon range of expertise and professional status. Whilst the provision and nature of learning support within Higher Education Institutions (HEIs) differs, the preferred model necessitates collaboration and integration across the institution, promoting independence. Despite models of good practice reinforcing and encouraging this approach (Association of Dyslexia Specialists in Higher Education, 2004), within many universities the model of support for students identified with a SpLD in the UK relies largely on funding through the Disabled Students Allowance (DSA).

Information processing

Understanding the way that information is processed may help to explain the challenges and difficulties faced by dyslexic individuals. There are three main

Table 34.1 Assessment framework

Assessment process	What happens	Intervention	Issues
Step 1 Obtain educational and family history Administer specific dyslexia screening test Other: handwriting and/or visual sensitivity	Initial findings and recommendations discussed with student including profile of individual strengths and weaknesses. Referral made for diagnostic assessment	Initial liaison and collaboration with departments Consider availability of generic intervention (study skills) Advice given regarding access to funding for the assessment Student continues to access generic study skills with progress monitored Further structured support is considered once assessment completed	*Note these are identified student concerns which may occur at any stage Disclosure Data protection and confidentiality Self esteem Course content (can I do this?) Motivation Placement issues Student role, responsibility (ownership) Managing dyslexia Impact of relationships (peers/ academic/ support staff)
Step 2 Student to apply for internal funding for full diagnostic assessment	Once funding approved, appointment with diagnostic assessor		
Step 3 Diagnostic assessment to determine: Cognitive ability Literacy skills Phonological skills	Full report sent to individual/institution Results and recommendations discussed with student, including proposed reasonable adjustments		
Step 4 Student to apply for external funding to support studies (Disabled Student Allowance) Reasonable adjustments developed (with student consent)	Appointment made for individual assessment of support needs Reasonable adjustments plan distributed to relevant persons confirming SpLD	Human and technological strategies of support agreed Reasonable adjustments implemented by university	
Step 5 Preparation of individual learning plan (in negotiation with student)	Student can access 1:1 specialist support Regular monitoring and review of needs	Specialist tuition to develop independent strategies of support Encourage use of assistive software	

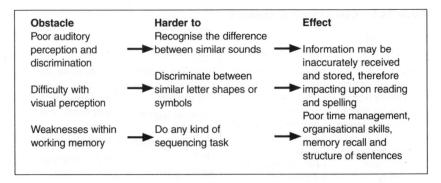

Obstacle	Harder to	Effect
Poor auditory perception and discrimination →	Recognise the difference between similar sounds →	Information may be inaccurately received and stored, therefore
Difficulty with visual perception →	Discriminate between similar letter shapes or symbols →	impacting upon reading and spelling
Weaknesses within working memory →	Do any kind of sequencing task →	Poor time management, organisational skills, memory recall and structure of sentences

Figure 34.1 Information processing cause and effect (adapted from DfES, 2005)

processes involved in learning – encoding, storage and retrieval – and information received is quickly lost unless a conscious effort is made to remember and transfer it to long-term memory (DfES, 2005). Inherent within the processing system are a number of obstacles or barriers, which generally affect the speed at which a task is completed, therefore making it more challenging (Figure 34.1).

Price (2004) considers the impact on working memory when processing and assimilating information, recognising the competition that exists for capacity to actually do 'the task'. If working memory is a weakness then a system of strategies is essential in order to reduce memory overload. However, as Cooper recognizes, 'many dyslexic learners still hide their difficulties, making it difficult to develop strategies to overcome the barriers', further emphasising the importance of that wider perspective (2009: 67).

Metacognition and learning

All students need a degree of metacognition to succeed academically and also improve self awareness and academic self concept (Gosling, 2003; Morgan, 2003). Dyslexic students need to acquire these metacognitive skills and awareness of strategies essential to effective and efficient learning at an early phase. Exploring how they learn should be part of planning, monitoring and appraising their own learning, to enhance and improve it. As knowledge further expands it is important to develop effective coping strategies by teaching students *how* to learn, not simply *what* to learn (McKay, 2004). However, learning is flexible and understanding patterns of behaviour and awareness of own learning style must encompass this in order to facilitate development (Mortimore, 2003).

CASE STUDY

Sam is a pre-registration nurse in the second year of a BSc in Adult Nursing. During the first year of her studies she achieved average marks of 40–48%

with feedback from tutors commonly noting inconsistency in spelling (particularly with the use of homophones) and poorly constructed sentences. Sam said she:

- has difficulty getting her thoughts down on paper and easily forgets.
- uses familiar words she can spell, rather than more complex vocabulary.
- has to read and re-read text slowly to try to understand meaning, which is time-consuming and tiring, particularly when she is on placement.

In addition, recording of information on placement was problematic due to written inaccuracies and slow speed of writing although placement mentors viewed Sam as an extremely diligent and personable student, holding a natural rapport with both staff and patients. Sam had been advised to seek support to enhance her academic skills but as yet she has not done so.

This case study illustrates typical characteristics that may indicate a student has an underlying difficulty that is impacting upon study and employment – but a balance has to be maintained. Whilst the importance of developing relationships across institutional and professional boundaries is central to enhancing availability of support, Sam herself also has to take ownership within this process; 'the dyslexic nurse must recognise in the first place that there are learning difficulties and seek assessment and support' (Dale and Aiken, 2007: 72).

How can Sam be supported?

- Adopt a proactive anticipatory approach in line with legislative and institutional guidelines.
- Work collaboratively and seek advice from specialists within support departments.
- Consider the use of grids and templates within the context of subject area to support weaker skills in the individual student and promote empowerment (Mortimore and Crozier, 2006; Price and Gale, 2006; Stainer and Ware, 2006).
- Follow good practice guidelines for lectures, seminars, accessibility and so forth; clarity of instruction and the way information is presented are crucial in teaching and learning and even more so when there are sequencing difficulties involved.
- Be clear and explicit (visually and verbally); making meaningful connections is essential for dyslexic learners and reinforces understanding and supports memory deficits (DfES, 2005).
- Work in manageable chunks, leaving time for processing and assimilation of information.

CONCLUSION

The degree and impact of dyslexia on the individual varies, necessitating a diversity of teaching methods, strategies and interventions, all requiring effective collaboration. The difficulties associated with a SpLD are not isolated or solely restricted to spelling, reading and writing, but also include emotional and psychological considerations, which impact upon a range of skills and tasks operating across all learning processes. It is vital to develop metacognitive awareness within the framework of a student's own learning, as dyslexic individuals need to attach meaning and take responsibility for their learning. Furthermore, as professionals, it is imperative that we are mindful of the importance of adopting that wider perspective if we are to fully partake in the inclusion process.

See also: assessment; dealing with failing and problem students; diversity and equality; study skills

FURTHER READING

Dale, C. and Aiken, F. (2007) *A Review of the Literature into Dyslexia in Nursing Practice.* Retrieved from Royal College of Nursing website: http://www.rcn.org.uk

Pollak, D. (ed.) (2009) *Neurodiversity in Higher Education: Positive Responses to Specific Learning Differences.* West Sussex: Wiley–Blackwell.

REFERENCES

Association of Dyslexia Specialists in Higher Education (2004) *Guidelines for Good Practice.* Retrieved from ADSHE website: http://adshe.org.uk/resources/

Cooper, R. (2009) 'Dyslexia', in D. Pollak (ed.), *Neurodiversity in Higher Education: Positive Responses to Specific Learning Differences.* West Sussex: Wiley– Blackwell. pp. 63–90.

Dale, C. and Aiken, F. (2007) *A Review of the Literature into Dyslexia in Nursing Practice.* Retrieved from Royal College of Nursing website: http://www.rcn.org.uk

Department for Education and Skills (2005) *Supporting Dyslexic Learners in Different Contexts.* Oxford: Nuffield Press.

Gosling, W. (2003) *Access to Higher Education for the Mature Dyslexic Student: A Question of Identity and a New Perspective.* Cascade Forum.

Jamieson, C. and Morgan, E. (2008) *Managing Dyslexia at University: A Resource for Students, Academic and Support Staff.* London: Routledge.

McKay, N. (2004) 'Success comes in cans, not can'ts – accelerating learning for dyslexic learners in the mainstream classroom through metacognition and emotional intelligence', in *On Dyslexia: The Dividends from Research to Practice* [CD]. Oldham: Inclusive Technology Ltd.

Morgan, E. (2003) 'The dyslexic adult in a non-dyslexic institution: making HE more dyslexia-friendly', in D. Pollak (ed.), *Supporting the Dyslexic Student in HE and FE: Strategies for Success.* Leicester: De Montfort University. pp. 20–35.

Mortimore, T. (2003) *Dyslexia and Learning Style: A Practitioner's Handbook.* London: Whurr Publishers.

Mortimore, T. and Crozier, W.R. (2006) 'Dyslexia and difficulties with study skills in Higher Education', *Studies in Higher Education,* 31 (2): 235–51.

Office for Disability Issues (2006) The Disability Equality Duty. Retrieved from Direct Gov website:www.direct.gov.uk/en/DisabledPeople/RightsAndObligations/DisabilityRights DG_1003105

Office of Public Sector Information (2005) Disability Discrimination Act. Retrieved from Direct Gov website: www.direct.gov.uk/en/DisabledPeople/EducationAndTraining/DG_ 4001076

Price, G.A. (2004) *The Dyslexic Cognitive Profile Linked to Compensatory Measures Adopted for Macro and Micro Text Generation by Dyslexic Undergraduate and Postgraduate Students*

key concepts in healthcare education

in HE. Paper presented at 6th BDA International Conference 2004. Retrieved from www. bdainternationalconference.org/2004/presentations/sun_s4_c_8.shm

Price, G.A. and Gale, A. (2006) 'How do dyslexic nursing students cope with clinical practice placements? The impact of the dyslexic profile on the clinical practice of dyslexic nursing students: pedagogical issues and considerations', *Learning Disabilities: A Contemporary Journal*, 4 (1): 19–36.

Reid, G. and Kirk, J. (2001) *Dyslexia in Adults: Education and Employment*. West Sussex: John Wiley and Sons.

Richardson, J. and Wydell, TN. (2003) 'The representation and attainment of students with dyslexia in UK Higher Education', *Reading and Writing: An Interdisciplinary Journal*, 16 (5): 475–503.

Stainer, L. and Ware, P. (2006) *Guidelines to Support Nursing Learners with Dyslexia in Practice*. Retrieved from ADSHE website: http://adshe.org.uk/wpcontent/uploads/good_practice_consultation1.pdf

Tinklin, T., Riddell, S. and Wilson, A. (2002) *Disabled Students in Higher Education: The Impact of Anti-Discrimination Legislation on Teaching, Learning and Assessment, Reconfiguring Sociology of Education*. University of Bristol: EScalate.

White, J. (2007) 'Supporting nursing students with dyslexia in clinical practice', *Nursing Standard*, 21 (19): 35–42.

35 student support

Annette McIntosh and Janice Gidman

DEFINITION

The term support comes from the Latin *supportare*, deriving from the term *portare*, meaning 'to carry'. The dictionary definition of support covers a wide range of applications, but the ones most pertinent to the concept of student support include the notions of giving assistance, encouragement or approval (Oxford English Dictionary, 2009). In healthcare education, the term refers to personal, academic and professional support in both university and practice settings.

KEY POINTS

- Effective support aids the retention and progression of students.
- Student support should be an integral part of healthcare programmes.
- The notion of student support is complex and there is a range of strategies to provide support in academic and practice settings.

DISCUSSION

The issue of student retention is a high priority for governments internationally (Zepke and Leach, 2005), especially with the on-going drive towards widening participation in Higher Education (HE). In the United Kingdom a recent Parliamentary Select Committee reported that, in order to achieve wider participation in HE, a comprehensive system of student support should be provided in addition to academic support; this incorporated pastoral care and welfare and strategies such as counselling, mentoring and pre-admission courses (Innovation, Universities, Science and Skills Committee, 2009).

Increasing attention is therefore being directed towards the need to develop and optimise student support in order to maximise achievement and minimise attrition. There are many factors that can contribute to enhancing student support, especially within healthcare provision, which includes pre-qualifying, post-qualifying and postgraduate programmes. In addition, as Jeffreys (2007) noted, students in healthcare, especially nursing programmes, come from a wide age range, with differing social and educational backgrounds and thus have diverse needs in relation to the support required to succeed in their studies. It is also the case that many students have to balance academic study with the development of professional competence and integration into practice areas.

The issue of student support has to be considered at the outset in the development of new programmes. In the approval of new provision, the sources and level of support for students should be clearly articulated, with evidence of the effective provision of the necessary mechanisms and resources, both human and physical. In recruiting students, and prior to their admission, there are various elements of support to be addressed, including financial aspects, diagnosing specific learning needs where possible and ensuring that students are supported in making the right choice of programme for them, through providing full and accurate information about the educational provision on offer.

In the delivery of healthcare programmes, it is the HE Institution's (HEI's) responsibility, often in tandem with clinical partners, to ensure that students are supported according to their individual needs, expectations and their level of study on an on-going basis.

Support can be provided from a range of diverse sources, summarised in Table 35.1, which demonstrates the complex and multi-factorial nature of supporting students in healthcare education. Hill et al. (2003) showed that students' perceptions of quality in HE included a positive learning atmosphere, the provision of social and emotional support systems, addressing such elements as childcare, peer networks and a student support unit. This study also highlighted the importance of readily available library and IT resources. Similarly, Robbins et al. (2004) stated that many factors contribute to student success, including the perceived social support and academic engagement within the HEI.

Smith (2007) opined that lecturing staff are best placed to provide the nurturing and individual support that students need in the academic setting, although increasing workloads and the adoption of the model of students as independent learners can make the development of meaningful, supportive

Table 35.1 Examples of common sources for student support

Academic	Practice	Overarching
• Personal tutors • Programme and module leaders • Programme administrators • Peers • Students' Union	• Mentors • Practice education facilitators • Clinical staff, including managers and health assistants • Peers • Link/personal tutors from HEI	• Family • Friends • Financial advice • Chaplaincy
HEI services such as: • Student support unit • Counsellors • Learning support unit • IT support		

relationships between students and academic staff challenging. Support from lecturers can range from tutorial support, either on subject-specific aspects or more generic elements such as academic writing skills, the latter often in conjunction with specialised support staff, to a more personalised, pastoral role. Gidman (2001) stated that three commonly agreed aspects of the personal tutor role in healthcare concerned academic, pastoral and clinical support roles.

Peer support and mentoring, both in academic and clinical settings, has been shown to be effective in the education of healthcare students. Aston and Molassiotis (2003) reported that peer support systems in practice, where senior students supervised junior students, enhanced motivation and helped reduce the anxieties of clinical practice, with the caveat that this required careful selection of capable and appropriate senior students for the role. Gilmour et al. (2007) noted that such schemes also have benefits for the personal and professional development of the student mentors, but cautioned that the mentees had to be adequately prepared and have clear expectations of the role and scope of the student mentor.

Support within practice settings is key for healthcare students, especially given that integration and socialisation processes can be very stressful. Recent attention has been paid to the concept of emotional intelligence, defined as a range of emotional and social competences necessary for success in daily life and the workplace (Benson et al., 2009). Montes-Berges and Augusto (2007) reported that healthcare students who were aware of, and heeded, their emotions were likely to rely on a coping strategy involving social support to deal with stressors and that it was important to prepare students accordingly. Brown and Edelmann (2000) showed that the most frequently reported stressors for healthcare students, in this case nurses, were achieving an appropriate work/life balance and financial anxieties, and that the highest degree of support came from the mentor, family, friends and peers.

Much has been written about the crucial role of the mentor in supporting students in practice. Cope et al. (2000) reported that a scaffolding approach supported learning in placements, whereby the level of support from mentors is gradually withdrawn as the competence, independence and confidence of the students increased. Caldwell et al. (2008) proposed a team mentoring model to offer a solid framework of support for students. The development of support roles involving experienced staff, such as practice educators, is also gaining momentum to supplement mentorship and the link lecturing roles of academics.

An important element in the concept of student support is listening to the views of the students themselves through consultation and evaluation systems and gaining feedback on the effectiveness of support mechanisms and ideas for improvement or innovation. HEIs should be proactive in this respect, enhancing support by listening and responding to the student voice and experience.

CASE STUDY

Ana is a midwifery student in the third year of her programme. She has a partner and two young children and she also works as a part-time healthcare assistant in a nursing home. She finds the workload on the programme to be extremely challenging – trying to balance practice experience, assignment preparation, work commitments and running a home. She has considered leaving the programme on several occasions but is determined to complete it because of her commitment to becoming a midwife. Ana has accessed a range of individuals for support during the programme:

- at home – her mother and sister have helped with childcare, her partner and close friend have listened and provided emotional support after particularly stressful shifts on placement.
- in the midwifery unit – her mentor and fellow students have helped her to reflect on her experiences and the manager has been flexible in relation to her shift pattern.
- in university – her personal academic tutor has helped her to balance the demands of practice and academic assignments, module leaders have provided support and constructive feedback on her work and her peers have provided moral support throughout.

Ana readily admits that without this support she would not have been able to complete the programme and her experience highlights the complex and essential nature of both informal and formal support networks for students on professional programmes.

CONCLUSION

It is evident that student support is an essential component in education, especially given the current political drivers in HE, such as widening participation and enhancing progression and achievement. Students in healthcare often have complex support needs, given the requirements to achieve both academically and clinically, alongside family and personal responsibilities. Support mechanisms include a wide range of strategies and involve lecturers, academic support staff and practitioners, along with the student's network of peers, family and friends. Clearly, healthcare educators need to have a strong commitment to the notion of student support and be competent in using appropriate strategies to this end.

See also: dealing with failing and problem students; feedback and marking; learning environments; mentorship; practice teaching; specific learning needs of students; study skills

FURTHER READING

Fry, H., Ketteridge, S. and Marshall, S. (2009) *A Handbook for Teaching and Learning in Higher Education*, 3rd edn. London: Routledge.

Responding to Student Need. Student Evaluation and Feedback Toolkit. www.enhancement-themes.ac.uk/documents/studentneeds/Student_Needs_Full_Outcomes_FINAL29_6_05.pdf

REFERENCES

Aston, L. and Molassiotis, A. (2003) 'Supervising and supporting student nurses in clinical practice: the peer support initiative', *Nurse Education Today*, 23 (3): 202–10.

Benson, G., Ploeg, J. and Brown, B. (2009) 'A cross-sectional study of emotional intelligence in baccalaureate nursing students', *Nurse Education Today*, 30 (1): 49–53.

Brown, H. and Edelmann, R. (2000) 'Project 2000: a study of expected and experienced stressors and support reported by students and qualified nurses', *Journal of Advanced Nursing*, 31 (4): 857–64.

Caldwell, J., Dodd, K. and Wilkes, C. (2008) 'Developing a team mentoring model', *Nursing Standard*, 23 (7): 35–9.

Cope, P., Cuthbertson, P. and Stoddart, B. (2000) 'Situated learning in the practice placement', *Journal of Advanced Nursing*, 31 (4): 850–6.

Gidman, J. (2001) 'The role of the personal tutor: a literature review', *Nurse Education Today*, 21 (5): 359–65.

Gilmour, J.A., Kopeikin, A. and Douche, J. (2007) 'Student nurse and peer-mentors: collegiality in practice', *Nurse Education in Practice*, 7 (1): 36–43.

Hill, Y., Lomas, L. and MacGregor, J. (2003) 'Students' perceptions of quality in higher education', *Quality Assurance in Higher Education*, 11 (1): 15–20.

Innovation, Universities, Science and Skills Committee (2009) *Students and Universities. Eleventh Report of Session 2008–09. Volume 1*. London: House of Commons.

Jeffreys, M.R. (2007) 'Non-traditional students' perceptions of variables influencing retention', *Nurse Educator*, 32 (4): 161–67.

Montes-Berges, B. and Augusto, J.M. (2007) 'Exploring the relationship between perceived and emotional intelligence, coping, social support and mental health in nursing students', *Journal of Psychiatric and Mental Health Nursing*, 14 (2): 163–71.

Oxford English Dictionary (2009) Retrieved from OED website: www.askoxford.com

Robbins, S.B., Lauver, K., Le, H., Davis, D. and Langley, R. (2004) 'Do psychosocial and study skill factors predict college outcomes? A meta-analysis', *Psychological Bulletin*, 130 (2): 261–88.

Smith, R. (2007) 'An overview of research on student support: helping students to achieve or achieving institutional targets? Nurture or de-nature?', *Teaching in Higher Education*, 12 (5): 683–95.

Zepke, N. and Leach, L. (2005) 'Integration and adaptation – approaches to the student retention and achievement puzzle', *Active Learning in Higher Education*, 6 (46): 46–59.

36 study skills

Elizabeth Mason-Whitehead

DEFINITION

Study skills is a generic term that refers to a wide range of strategies and approaches that can be applied to the process of learning. Studying is an experience that should be seen as a dynamic and on-going process that is inextricably linked to lifelong learning.

Our starting point is that 'education deals with students as people, who are diverse in all respects, and ever changing' (Fry et al., 2003: 1).

KEY POINTS

- Students have a very wide range of backgrounds, abilities, experiences and ages and their study needs may be correspondingly different. Students with specific learning difficulties must be acknowledged, supported and given equal opportunities.
- Study skills include managing time and self-directed study effectively, developing critical thinking strategies, understanding technology and accessing and using literature.
- Students need to convey the theoretical underpinnings to a practical application, particularly in relation to professional programmes. Students in healthcare are frequently asked to reflect upon their practice; understanding models and theories of reflection are therefore essential study skills.

DISCUSSION

Why do students continue to struggle with essay construction, accurate referencing and preparing for examinations when Higher Education Institutions (HEIs) are awash with study skills material? The answer is probably found in a range of areas, including students not taking study skills seriously, a miscalculated belief that everything will be alright and an underestimation of the level of academic performance required to be successful. All students (and lecturers!) require a basic set of study skills to pursue their academic studies. Figure 36.1 is intended to help students ascertain their baseline study skill strengths and those areas requiring further development.

We will now discuss in more detail these fundamental study skills and particularly those that cause the most concern.

My study skill area	I attended lecturer/ teaching session	I require/ do not require further support	Particular challenges	Plans for development
Time management	Attended time management session 30/09/09	Require more support	Find it difficult to manage studies and child care and I am often late for lectures and do not submit my assignments in on time	1 Arranged meeting with PAT 2 Planned meeting with Student Support Officer 3 Place offered for children in university nursery
Self directed learning				
Special learning needs				
Information technology				
Referencing: Harvard/ APA/Vancouver				
Assignment writing				
Preparing for written examinations				
Preparing for other examinations				
Relating Theory to practice				
Other study skill areas identified by student/ course/lecturer heavier rule				

Figure 36.1   Study skill self assessment and action plan

Know Yourself

Knowing yourself is a fundamental prerequisite to successful studying. Asking students to take time to understand what kind of student they are and developing their 'weaker' areas will ultimately pay dividends. The following questions will prompt students to explore and reflect on their study skills:

- Do they ever avoid studying?
- What are their avoidance strategies for studying (for example, cleaning out cupboards or washing their car)?
- Do they feel uncomfortable showing someone else their written work or become overly anxious before exams?
- Do they lack confidence with spelling or reading?

If students answer 'yes' to any of these questions they can be reassured that they are not alone and that these anxieties can be readily addressed.

Special Needs

Some students find the term being 'labelled' a person with 'special educational needs' stigmatising (Mason-Whitehead and Mason, 2008) and are dissuaded from entering university because they fear that their special needs will obstruct their academic progress. However, students joining Higher Education (HE) today have never been better placed to have their special needs identified and supported.

Managing Time

Whatever stage we are at in our careers, managing time remains one of the greatest challenges. Many people are overwhelmed by the number of competing demands for their time, which may prompt them not to commence or complete their chosen programme of study. However, with some careful planning it is amazing what can be achieved! Students who often feel under the greatest stress are those who express concerns that their families don't understand the academic input that is required. Take, for example, a mother of two children undertaking a nursing degree. Although she has her childcare organised, she still requires support from her family which will allow her to study. Such a student typically reports to her Personal Academic Tutor (PAT) that her family will ask why she needs so much study time. The chart in Figure 36.2 is intended to be created not only by the student but shared with the significant people in his or her life, and therefore the studying process becomes a joint venture between all the family members.

Information Technology

We often make the assumption that we inhabit a world where everyone lives and breathes computers. However, lecturers teaching study skills will quickly realise that the level of information technology competence amongst any given group of students is very varied, with some being able to set up websites and others struggling to find the on/off button! This very uneven playing field can give rise to considerable anxiety amongst some students. Reassurance, guidance and support in developing students' skills in information technology are critical to their overall development and an area in which HEIs have a fundamental role to play.

Time	Monday	Tuesday	Wednesday	Thursday	Friday	Saturday	Sunday
MORNING							
6–7		Study				Study	
7–8	Early shift			Early shift			
8–9	Winston doing school run	School run	Study Winston to do school run	Emma to do school run	School run		
9–10					Research assignment subsmission 9.30	Clare: hockey, take sandwiches for 30	
10–11					David: hospital appointment 10.30		
11–12							
AFTERNOON							
12–1			Study		Late shift	David: football	Parents' lunch
1–2			Study				
2–3			Study				
3–4	Winston: School run		Winston: school run	Emma: school run	Winston: school run and tea		
4–5	David: Dentist 5 pm	Clare: Piano 4.30					
EVENING							
5–6	Poppy for tea	David and Clare at Sue's for tea					
6–7		Study					
7–8	Clare: Parent's Evening 7.30	Study				Family dinner	
8–9	Study	Study	Study	Study			Study
9–10							
10–11							
11–12							

Week beginning October 5th 2009

Figure 36.2 Weekly time management plan

Managing Literature and Related Material

Many lecturers and students entering academia are overwhelmed by the abundance of literature from which to draw and this challenge cannot be ignored. The reasons are two-fold; firstly, literature forms the basis of the evidence which supports and guides clinical practice, and secondly, literature is fundamental to HE and as the health professions develop so does the literature; this is a benchmark by which we judge our place within any given discipline.

The starting point for managing literature is the library and accompanying learning resources departments of the HEI. Many librarians provide excellent tutorials on accessing literature and using resources, such as databases. Libraries can be intimidating places and it always appears that other students know what they are doing – they often don't! But what people are doing is familiarising themselves with one of the most important places in the HEI and the more time students spend in the library, becoming increasingly confident with literature searches, using journals, databases and so forth, the greater the evidence they will have for assignments and other assessments.

Assignment Writing

Writing remains the universal criterion by which a great number of programmes within HE are assessed. The fear of writing is also a reason for considerable anxiety amongst lecturers and students alike. However, once someone begins writing, with appropriate support, the experience can be not only rewarding but life-changing. Approaching assignment writing in the same way as addressing other study skills, in a step-by-step method, can reduce the perceived insurmountable task to an achievable objective, as explained in Figure 36.3.

Concept mapping

Concept mapping has proved to be one of the most effective strategies in critical thinking (Gul and Borman, 2006). It is most useful in its application to practice as it engages students in decision-making. The actual map is made up of circles or cells, with the central concept or question in the centre with lines or links to other cells to show the relationships. These free associations are exercises that help solve problems and bring students together and can be used within study groups. The value of working in small groups can often be a safe haven for mutual support and cohesion (Overton et al., 2009).

Referencing

Referencing is the 'necessary evil' of studying and writing. If a student decides that referencing is a waste of time and has nothing to do with what they want to do, then university is not for them. Referencing serves two main purposes:

Stage of assignment	Date commenced	Completed date	Additional notes
Stage 1: Assignment details	Date assignment details given: Word length: Question/area to be addressed:		
Stage 2: Preparation phase			Note: the assignment submission date is the day of David's hospital appointment Library work
Stage 3: Writing phase Dividing the assignment into sections will make the assignment less daunting	Literature search Title Abstract Introduction Literature review Discussion References Printing/submission		

Figure 36.3   Assignment writing plan

it supports the argument that is being made and it allows the reader to check and follow up statements.

Just as accurate referencing informs the reader that the author is academically mature, referencing that is incorrect is a sign that the author produces work that is sloppy and unprofessional. Furthermore, writing that is copied and not referenced is plagiarism. This is an 'academic crime', invoking the academic malpractice policy within the HEI that can lead to a range of penalties, of which expulsion from the programme is the most severe.

There are four commonly used referencing systems: Legal, Vancouver, American Psychological Association (APA) and Harvard. For students and academics working in healthcare, the last three are the most commonly used. Referencing is an on-going learning process and Figure 36.4 charts a student's referencing progress.

Guided study and self-directed learning (SDL)

How many student timetables include sessions on guided study or SDL? Probably most weekly timetables will have one such slot, but what does it mean to the student? An afternoon in the library? An opportunity to catch up with the laundry, perhaps? With some explanation and support, both guided study and SDL can be positive experiences that enhance study skills. Indeed,

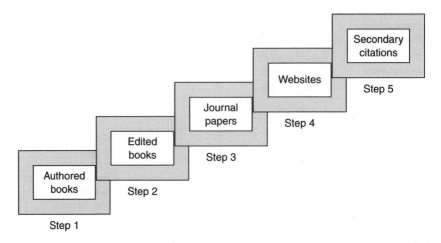

Figure 36.4 Steps to successful referencing

Move up the steps as you become more competent with referencing, authored books
being the easiest and secondary citations the most difficult.
The steps can be used to monitor your progress on each type of referencing, e.g. APA.

the evidence suggests that students only engage with SDL when they are
given specific guidance and feedback from their work (Regan, 2003). A
fundamental prerequisite for SDL is the student's readiness and preference
for this form of study (O'Shea, 2003) and some students will take longer to
reach this point. For those students who have reached academic maturity,
SDL has many benefits, including increased confidence, autonomy, motivation
and the preparation for lifelong learning (O'Shea, 2003).

CASE STUDY

David, a 34-year-old restaurant manager, had a long-standing ambition to
become a nurse in a hospital Accident and Emergency Department. However,
David's negative experiences of studying at school left him so traumatised he
was unable to pursue any academic qualifications, until his younger cousin
Sophie, started her health degree at the local HEI. Sophie had been diagnosed
with dyslexia at school and was offered assistance from the HEI's Student
Support Unit together with one-to-one tutorials with her Personal Academic
Tutor. After some persuasion from Sophie, David approached the HEI and
asked if he could be given guidance on working towards the qualifications
required for his chosen programme. It took some time for David to build up
his confidence, but he persevered with his studies and received a range of
study skill support. Today, David is in the third year of his nursing studies
degree and his dream of being an Accident and Emergency nurse is becoming
a reality.

CONCLUSION

This discussion has demonstrated that the experience of studying is considerably more complex than we would first imagine. As the case study illustrates, negative memories of school can have a profound impact on future educational encounters and be a source of both distress and anxiety. As educationalists and students we need to work to overcome these challenges. Ultimately, however, successful studying is rooted in the belief that learning is for life and that it should be enjoyed to the full.

See also: academic staff development; e-learning; information literacy; learning environments; learning styles; reflection; research and scholarly activity; specific learning needs of students; student support

FURTHER READING

Ridley, D. (2008) *The Literature Review. A Step-by-Step Guide for Students*. London: Sage.
Walliman, N. (2004) *Your Undergraduate Dissertation. The Essential Guide for Success*. London: Sage.

REFERENCES

Fry, H., Ketteridge, S. and Marshall, S. (2003) *A Handbook for Teaching and Learning in Higher Education*, 2nd edn. London: Kogan Page.
Gul, R.B. and Borman, J.A. (2006) 'Concept mapping: a strategy for teaching and evaluation in nursing education', *Nurse Education in Practice*, 6 (4): 199–206.
Mason-Whitehead, E. and Mason, T. (2008) *Study Skills for Nurses*, 2nd edn. London: Sage.
O'Shea, E. (2003) 'Self-directed learning in nurse education: a review of the literature', *Journal of Advanced Nursing*, 43: 63–70.
Overton, G.K., Kelly, D., McCallister, P., Jones, J. and Macvicar, R. (2009) 'The practice-based small group learning approach: making evidence-based practice come alive for learners', *Nurse Education Today*, 29 (6): 671–5.
Regan, J.A. (2003) 'Motivating students towards self-directed learning', *Nurse Education Today*, 23 (8): 593–9.

study skills

37 supervising masters and phd students

Tom Mason

If you want to know the way ahead, ask someone coming back (Old Chinese proverb)

DEFINITION

The academic educational process of supervision is grounded in the provision of a healthy environment in which growth and development can occur, experimentation and testing of the world safely is encouraged and evaluation and reflection is promoted. Through this process it is intended that the student will cultivate the ability to balance arguments based on the logic of science. Although students may require high dependency supervision in the early stages, this may 'loosen' as they mature into critical thinkers and gain in both knowledge and confidence. Supervision can be defined as overseeing, overlooking, watching-out for, guiding, supporting and encouraging someone with less experience in a particular area of life.

KEY POINTS

- Supervision is concerned with a professional academic relationship.
- Different expectations may exist between supervisor and student, which can lead to problems.
- Different levels of reading, understanding, critique, analysis and synthesis are evident between Masters and PhD study.
- Supervision aims may be different for the supervisor and the student.
- Different supervisory strategies need to be applied depending on the assessment of the student.

DISCUSSION

A review of the literature regarding the supervision of Masters and PhD programmes of research emphasises the point that success or failure tends to pivot on the *relationship* between the supervisor and the student, particularly with

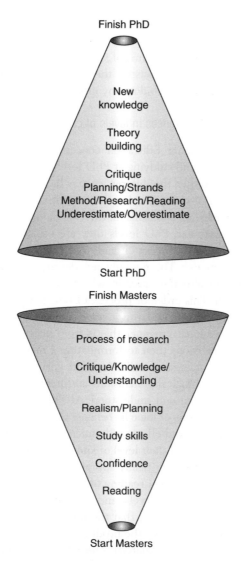

Figure 37.1   **Masters build up and PhD focus down 'journey'**

regard to the expectations that each has of the process, the content, their own
role and that of the other. Therefore, laying down these expectations with clarity and discussion early on in the process is vitally important for all concerned
on what is usually described as a 'journey'. It may be helpful to illustrate this
'journey' in terms of a funnel-shaped route (see Figure 37.1), with the Masters
programme building up and the PhD study focusing down. However, whilst
this main emphasis is placed on the relationship between the supervisor and the
student it should also be noted that there are other reasons for both success and
failure of the student. The following discussion will attempt to outline the

two-way process between supervisor and student by focusing on four specific and potentially problematic areas of supervision: differences in levels of critique; differences in expectations; aims of supervision; and supervision strategy. Hopefully, this will provide signposts for the 'journey', both in terms of safely arriving at the destination and avoiding any pitfalls along the way.

Differences in levels of critique

A common debate in Higher Education concerns the differences between studying at Masters level and studying at PhD level and, sadly, there is no one simple answer to this. Rather, the differences may be appreciated in a number of areas, with the level of critique being the first. Students' ability to critique relies on their knowledge of, and skills in, the area in which they are working. For example, at Masters and PhD levels they are usually, but by no means always, undertaking a piece of research and in this scenario they will need to know the process of research. This not only includes the right method to answer the right question but also the order in which the components of research should be undertaken. This order, or process, of research is based on the logic of scientific enquiry. Simply stated, this involves moving from one stage of the process to the next in a logical manner, that is, from reviewing the literature to identifying research questions then to formulating a method to answer those questions followed by accessing, collecting and analysing data from which results are produced and logical conclusions are drawn. At Masters level this process ought to be known and understood. At PhD level it should also be appreciated that the relations of logic lie *between* the stages of research, that is, the relation between cause and effect, and understanding and prediction.

Students' level of study and their level of knowledge of the research process will determine their ability to critically appraise their own method as well as other published research. Critical reading of other research is a central component of study at both these levels, and an expected difference between Masters and PhD critical reading is that the former may be limited to structure and content (that is, ensuring the production of the method comes after the research questions are formulated) whilst the latter may include challenges of the relations between the stages (that is, that a particular cause may not have produced the reported effect).

Differences in expectations

Expectations at Masters and PhD levels are often implicit rather than made explicit and herein lies the potential for problems. A starting point for analysing differences in expectations is the consideration of what may be termed 'supervision proximity'. This refers to the 'closeness' of the supervisor to the student in relation to what is going on in their study, their growth of knowledge and their abilities. As a general guide it is widely agreed that the supervisor proximity is closest at undergraduate level, becoming slightly more distant on Masters programmes and most distant on PhD studies. However, in reality it is not quite as simple as this, as supervisory proximity is dependent, again, on the individual knowledge, skills and abilities of each student. Furthermore, the proximity is often adjusted throughout a course of study in relation to the needs of the student at various stages.

Although supervisors' and students' expectations may differ, the central issues are the proximity of the relationship and knowing the areas of responsibilities. An exhaustive listing of roles and responsibilities is not feasible here, however, a brief outline of the most common ones may suffice. The expectation that the student will read is fundamental and at Masters level this reading should be comprehensive in the study area, whilst at PhD level it should be extensive and incorporate all material directly related to the study area as well as relevant literature in associated fields. The student is also expected to plan and execute their project. Whilst supervisors may offer guidance and support it is the responsibility of the student to engage with the planning and to do it themselves. A common conflict is concerned with the setting up and recording of supervision sessions. It is students' responsibility to arrange these sessions and to make their own record, however, supervisors may also be required to ensure that the supervision sessions take place and to make their own record of such meetings. Finally, at Masters level it is expected that the growth of students' knowledge and their ability to synthesise will develop without necessarily producing new knowledge or theory, whilst at PhD level this is a fundamental requirement (Marshall and Green, 2007).

Aims of supervision

The aims of supervision are of a dynamic quality, with some referring to the supervisor and some to the student. The main aim for the supervisor is to assess the progress of the student in relation to their level, be it Masters or PhD, and the stage which they are at on their programme. In practice, the supervisor is usually gathering further information relating to the student's knowledge base, critical ability, reading level as well as their enthusiasm, commitment and overall mental-set regarding their studies. Thus, the aims of the supervisor relate to the progress, growth and development of the student, geared towards their level of study.

Supervision aims also change in style over the course of Masters and PhD studies, with the early phases requiring a more teaching or 'telling them what to do' approach, which ought to develop into a guiding or suggesting style as the student progresses and gains confidence. The aims then move towards a support or 'asking them what they think they ought to do' approach, which leads on to a 'sounding board' or 'what are your options?' type of framework. Thus, the aims are closely related to the relationship between supervisor and student.

Supervision strategy

With the vagaries of human nature being as diverse as they are and the differences in personalities being wide, for both supervisors and students, it is not possible to set out one style of supervision nor one strategy that will fit all. However, the supervision strategy ought to be flexible and be able to respond to both the student's progress and the life events that impact on their study. In the assessment of the student supervision, the supervisor is appraising the abilities of the student to progress, which involves all the aspects mentioned above such as reading, planning, executing, critiquing, analysing, synthesising, and so on. Thus, there are two broad strategies of supervision that may be required in response to the assessment of the student and their level of study. These strategies can be termed 'hands off' and 'hands on'.

The 'hands off' strategy is usually employed in response to the student developing well, making good progress with their project, responding effectively to objectives that are set and achieving their goals accordingly. In this strategy the supervisor may observe from a distance through supervision sessions and let the student lead their studies within the confines of the programme timetable. Clearly this strategy involves a confidence in both the supervisor and the student that the study is going well and according to plan. However, this is not always the case and if the supervision assessment concludes that the student requires a closer style of supervision, possibly because of the weakness of the student, their poor planning and management, or events making execution of the project difficult, then a 'hands on' strategy may need to be developed. This may involve an increase in supervision meetings, regular contact, frequent early drafts or reports, specific feedback and straight-talking. In this approach it may be necessary to set the student short-term objectives with outcomes that can be measured or organise a reading programme with frequent discussions regarding a critique of the literature. This strategy may also involve specialist advice or remedial courses such as research methods, statistics or software training. If the student's response is positive then the 'hands on' strategy may be loosened a little – but the supervisor would be wise to keep a regular assessment of the student through supervision sessions (Rugg and Petre, 2004).

CASE STUDY

Following their PhD supervision sessions, Tony and Cristina had a coffee and swapped stories about their research projects. Tony complained about his supervisor, who seemed to change his mind every session and was constantly e-mailing Tony for updates. Tony showed Cristina the reading list and bemoaned how he was ever going to get through it all. He also expressed his concern about his knowledge of research methods and the fact that he did not have a Masters degree. Tony revealed that he had not even begun to think about his annual report and that he did not think a PhD was 'all it was cracked up to be'. Cristina was sympathetic but did not tell Tony that her studies were going well, that her Masters degree had prepared her for the PhD programme and that her supervisor was now letting her develop her studies using her own initiative. Cristina was excited that she was now beginning to believe that she would finally finish this 'journey'.

CONCLUSION

Each supervision relationship differs due to a number of factors. These include the personalities of both the supervisor and student, the nature of the expectations that each holds, the styles that are adopted and the breadth of expectations that both will bring to the experience. Finally, there are also different starting points for both the supervisor and the student with their varying levels of experience in their respective roles. It is advantageous to discuss these issues very early in the process rather than try to solve problems later as they occur.

See also: academic staff development; assessment; dealing with failing and problem students; mastery; mentorship; peer support and observation; reflection; research and scholarly activity; student support; study skills

FURTHER READING

Cryer, P. (2006) *The Research Student's Guide to Success*, 3rd edn. Maidenhead: Open University Press.

Murray, R. (2006) *How to Write a Thesis*, 2nd edn. Maidenhead: Open University Press.

Phillips, E. and Pugh, D.S. (2005) *How to Get a PhD: A Handbook for Students and their Supervisors*, 4th edn. Maidenhead: Open University Press.

REFERENCES

Marshall, S. and Green, N. (2007) *Your PhD Companion: A Handy Mix of Practical Tips, Sound Advice and Helpful Commentary to see you through your PhD*, 2nd edn. Oxford: How To Books Ltd.

Rugg, G. and Petre, M. (2004) *The Unwritten Rules of PhD Research*. Maidenhead: Open University Press.

supervising masters and phd students

38 teaching strategies

Jan Woodhouse

DEFINITION

A teaching strategy is an approach taken by the facilitator of learning that enables the aim of the session to be achieved. For example, if transfer of new knowledge is the aim then a short lecture might be delivered; on the other hand, if attitudes need to be explored then a debate may be used.

KEY POINTS

- There is a wide range of teaching strategies available.
- Teaching strategies in healthcare may change depending on the setting – classroom or practice.
- The choice of a teaching strategy can move the learner from being dependent to self directed.

DISCUSSION

The selection of an appropriate teaching strategy within healthcare education is important in order to maximise student learning. The term 'student' is used here in a very broad sense, that is, it could be a person on a programme of education or someone attending a one-off update session as part of their continuing professional development (CPD).

Range of teaching strategies

There are several elements to consider when choosing a teaching strategy. The starting points are the aims and objectives for the session: if the aim is to impart new knowledge to students then the strategy may include, for part of the session, a lecture; if you are seeking to change attitudes, then a hearty debate may be the core strategy;or if you want the person to try out a practical skill, simulation may be adopted. So the domain you are trying address in your aims and objectives, be it the cognitive, affective or psychomotor domain, will alter the teaching strategy. Healthcare education usually demands engagement with all of the domains and subsequently the students should encounter a range of strategies.

There are several writers on education who have evaluated or tabulated the range of teaching strategies available (Reece and Walker, 2000; Scales, 2008; Woodhouse, 2007a). Table 38.1 indicates the range of teaching strategies commonly discussed, plus additional strategies encountered by the author. The choice of strategy may depend on the number of students attending a session. The strategies are followed by the letters LG, indicating suitability for teaching large groups (more than 20), SG for small groups (5 to 20), or I for individuals (less than 5).

Table 38.1   The range of teaching strategies

- Lecture (LG)
- Discussion (LG)
- Demonstration (LG)
- Questions and answers (LG)
- Panel (LG)
- Team teaching (LG)
- Storytelling (LG)
- Blended and e-learning (LG)
- Film and video (LG)
- Podcast (LG)
- Radio and TV programmes (LG)
- Debate (LG)
- Idea storming (also known as brainstorming, thought or word showers, green hat thinking) (LG)
- Group work/buzz groups (SG)
- Simulation (SG)
- Case study (SG)
- Role-play (SG)
- Games and quizzes (SG)
- Sharing circle (SG)
- Visualisations (SG)
- Ice-breaker (SG)
- Experiential exercises (SG)
- Narratives (SG)
- Creative arts (SG)
- Seminars (SG)
- Field trips (SG)
- Body awareness (SG)
- Laboratory/workshop (SG)
- Problem-based learning [PBL] (SG/I)
- Scenario-generated learning [SGL] (SG/I)
- Presentations (SG/I)
- Concept mapping (SG/I)
- Discovery learning (SG/I)
- Supervision time (in group or one-to-one) (SG/I)
- Projects (I)
- Coaching (I)
- Reflection (I)
- Tutorials (I)
- Micro-teaching (I)
- Guided study (I)
- Self-directed study (I)
- Open/distance learning (I)

Sources: Kiger, 2004; Quinn and Hughes, 2007; Reece and Walker, 2000; Scales, 2008; Woodhouse, 2007a

This plethora of strategies indicates the desire of educators to offer the student a meaningful learning experience. Even within a teaching strategy, such as group work, there are additional ways of organising the session. Keen (2007), for example, cites the use of cross-over groups, fish-bowl groups and tutor-less groups, whilst Quinn and Hughes (2007) outline the use of syndicate groups, project groups, snowballing and carousel exercises. Similarly sessions with a communication focus, such as counselling skills, will use group work in the form of a sharing circle or as triads, where a group of three are split into client role, professional's role and observer role in order to practice their skills.

Depending on the length of a session the educator may use several teaching strategies, and Scales (2008) talks of the session having an introduction, development and an ending, likening it to a musical rhythm. The longer the intended session, the more likely it is that different teaching strategies will be used.

Learning in and from practice

Most of the strategies mentioned above are used in an education institution. However, for healthcare students, the environment where they make contact with the patient, client, relatives or other members of the multi-disciplinary team is a rich learning environment. Table 38.2 provides a list of teaching strategies that can be found and used in practice. Most of them will be directed at individual learning, although strategies such as demonstrations and opportunistic teaching can be addressed in a small group.

Table 38.2 Practice-based teaching strategies

• Interactions with patients, clients and relatives	• Reflective diaries/blogs
• History-taking	• Self-directed study
• Experiential learning	• Computer-aided learning
• Demonstration	• Ward rounds or home/clinic visits
• Observation	• Case study
• Opportunistic teaching	• Role modelling
• Questions and answers	• Simulation
• Critical incident review	• Narratives
• Audit and research	• Case conferences
• Handover reports	• Clinical supervision
• Skills practice	• Interactions with the multi-disciplinary team
• PBL	

Sources: Feather and Fry, 2009; Quinn and Hughes, 2007; Woodhouse, 2007b

Given the range of learning opportunities available in practice it is always surprising when you chance upon a student and, in response to asking what they have learned in their most recent placement, you receive the answer 'nothing'. How could they not have learned something? The answer to this conundrum is that the perception of their learning has often been clouded by a negative experience. The role models may have been poor, there might have been no opportunity to attend a vital demonstration, or there might have been a critical incident which has left the healthcare team upset and defensive of their practice. Subsequently, time has to pass before positive recollections can emerge.

From dependent to self-directed learner

Whilst you may have considered the domain in choosing your teaching strategy, there are other considerations. Think about who the students are – are they individuals with no knowledge of healthcare, who may consequently be very dependent on the educator? These dependent students may voice that they prefer lectures and demonstrations over other forms of teaching. If they are on a programme of study, then it is possible to develop the student to being self directed through the progressive use of different teaching strategies such as group presentations, small seminars, guided study and scenario-generated learning until they reach a stage of personal presentations, based on their own enquiries.

McHardy and Allan (2000) suggest that appreciation of skills and the underpinning knowledge are best served by conventional learning such as lectures, tutorials and directed reading. When applying the skills problem solving, case study analysis and projects (either individual or group) are most suited, whilst developing knowledge independently requires research or extended essays. Developing competence requires the use of intuitive and creative strategies, role-play, simulation, idea storming and fishbowling (McHardy and Allan, 2000). Education in the medical profession, for example, makes great use of problem-based learning (PBL) as a teaching strategy, which facilitates the individual to think like a doctor (Feather and Fry, 2009), that is, working as an autonomous practitioner. Dix and Hughes (2004) point out that students in healthcare come from a variety of backgrounds, cultures and age groups and as a result the educators need to be adaptable in their use of strategies, to meet the needs of the students.

The frequency with which an educator uses a strategy should also be borne in mind. One nursing student once commented to me: 'If I see another flip chart I shall scream!' She had obviously had too much of the group work strategy. Similarly, Feather and Fry (2009) comment that although medical students enjoy PBL they worry about whether they have learned enough to pass their assessments.

The relationship between teaching strategies and the role of education in health

The objective of education in health is to get to a point where the practitioner can operate safely, with the right knowledge, skills and attitudes in order to maintain the confidence of the patient or client. As such, many of the teaching strategies chosen will have the interpersonal as their focus – dealing with patients, clients, relatives and other members of the multi-disciplinary team. However, we must not forget the 'I' in the healthcare setting.

Having an understanding of ourselves, that is, knowledge of the intra-personal, can enhance the inter-personal aspects. Teaching strategies such as experiential exercises, body awareness and visualisations are directed at intra-personal knowledge – how do we feel, how do we react, what were we thinking when such and such happened? So, for example, we can use a lecture to deliver the stages of breaking bad news and make the assumption that, because the student has sat through the lecture and even discussed the issues with colleagues, that person will become effective at that skill. However intra-personal exploration may show that the individual lacks confidence or does not have the emotional resilience to deal with the potential backlash from the delivery of such news. Dix and Hughes (2004) note the value of reflection in the learning process, which could identify such intra-personal issues, and comment that students may need help with this, both in the classroom setting and in practice.

CASE STUDY

I recently attended a course entitled 'Healing through art'. We were a small group of mature students, from different parts of the world, numbering nine, including the facilitator. Each morning started with 15 minutes of directed study (drawing the same view/object). This was quickly followed by 10 minutes of bodywork, where we concentrated on our breathing and moving our limbs, sufficient to wake us all up. We then engaged in a sharing circle (to find out how each of us was feeling) before moving on to a brief demonstration (on the use of particular art materials) and a lengthy experiential exercise. After breaking during the experiential exercise for morning coffee, we returned to the exercise until lunch-time. In the afternoon we engaged with reflection to explore, with the others on the course, what emotions arose during the experiential exercise. This pattern of strategies was repeated over the next few days and at the end of the week we also shared the results of our directed study.

This case study shows that a variety of teaching strategies were used to facilitate learning at an intra-personal level, with a group of mature, motivated individuals. The activities were roughly in 20 minute time slots, but extra time was appropriately given for the experiential component. Where directed study had been given, time was allocated for feedback on the study.

CONCLUSION

It can be stated that there are many teaching strategies available to the facilitator of education. Knowledge of the students, and their development towards becoming self-directed learners, is essential in deciding what strategy to choose. For healthcare professionals, whose work involves a high level of underpinning knowledge, problem solving, teamwork, application of skills and interpersonal relationships, it is likely that all strategies will be used at some time during their education. It is therefore desirable that the facilitator of education is similarly familiar with the range of strategies and applies them appropriately.

See also: curriculum models and design; experiential and work-based learning; learning styles; practice teaching; reflection; role model; simulated learning and OSCEs; teaching styles

Reece, I. and Walker, S. (1997) *Teaching and Learning: A Practical Guide*, 3rd edn. Sunderland: Business Education Publishers.

Woodhouse, J. (ed.) (2007) *Strategies for Healthcare Education: How to Teach in the 21st Century*. Oxford: Radcliffe Medical.

REFERENCES

Dix, G. and Hughes, S.J. (2004) 'Strategies to help students learn effectively', *Nursing Standard*, 18 (32): 39–42.

Feather, A. and Fry, H. (2009) 'Key aspects of teaching and learning in medicine and dentistry', in H. Fry, S. Ketteridge and S. Marshall (eds), *A Handbook for Teaching and Learning in Higher Rducation*, 3rd edn. London: Routledge. pp. 424–48.

Keen, A. (2007) 'Small group learning: greater than the sum of its parts?', in J. Woodhouse (ed.), *Strategies for Healthcare Education: How to Teach in the 21st Century*. Oxford: Radcliffe Medical. pp. 17–27.

Kiger, A.M. (2004) *Teaching for Health*, 3rd edn. Edinburgh: Churchill Livingstone.

McHardy, P. and Allan, T. (2000) 'Closing the gap between what industry needs and what HE provides', *Education and Training*, 42 (9): 496–508.

Quinn, F.M. and Hughes, S.J. (2007) *Quinn's Principles and Practice of Nurse Education*, 5th edn. Cheltenham: Nelson Thornes.

Reece, I. and Walker, S. (2000) *Teaching and Learning: A Practical Guide*, 4th edn. Sunderland: Business Education Publishers.

Scales, P. (2008) *Teaching in the Lifelong Learning Sector*. Maidenhead: Open University Press.

Woodhouse, J. (ed.) (2007a) *Strategies for Healthcare Education: How to Teach in the 21st Century*. Oxford: Radcliffe Medical.

Woodhouse, J. (2007b) 'Applying strategies to practice', in J. Woodhouse (ed.), *Strategies for Healthcare Education: How to Teach in the 21st Century*. Oxford: Radcliffe Medical. pp. 135–44.

39 teaching styles

Janice Gidman with case study by Mark Hellaby

DEFINITION

There is no clear definition of the term 'teaching styles' in the education literature and the term is often used interchangeably with 'teaching strategies' and 'teaching methods'. Jarvis (2006) contends that the concept of teaching style recognises that the lecturer's performance is an integral aspect of the teaching process, proposing that 'style is about the art of teaching rather than the science. It is also about the teacher's own humanity and personality' (2006: 24). Jarvis also reports that there is considerable overlap between teaching styles and strategies, since the lecturer normally selects methods that are consistent with his/her personality. However, Jarvis maintains that teaching styles and methods are distinct concepts - for example it is possible to be a democratic lecturer or an autocratic facilitator.

KEY POINTS

- There is currently no commonly accepted definition of teaching styles.
- Teaching styles are influenced by the personal and philosophical stance of the lecturer.
- Teaching styles need to be appropriate for the content of the session and the nature of the group of students.
- Creativity and humour can enhance student learning.
- Lecturers should develop a range of teaching styles to meet the requirements of professional programmes in healthcare.

DISCUSSION

Effective teaching

Biggs and Tang (2007) advise that effective lecturers enable deep approaches to learning and support students to achieve their learning outcomes. They ensure that outcomes, content, assessment and teaching methods are constructively aligned and establish a learning climate which optimises interactions with their students. This student-centred approach involves an equal relationship between lecturer and student, which is encapsulated in the seminal work of Paulo Freire:

> The role of the educator is not to 'fill' the educatee with 'knowledge', technical or otherwise. It is rather to attempt to move towards a new way of thinking in both educator and educatee, through the dialogical relationships between both. (Freire, [1974]2005: 112)

However, student-centred learning approaches to teaching and learning require increased time and commitment from lecturers, mentors and practice educators and they require considerable skill to facilitate students' abilities to become self directed in their learning. Sander et al. (2000) explored undergraduate students' expectations and preferences in relation to teaching, learning and assessment. They concluded that, although students expected formal lectures, they reported that these were ineffective and their preference was for interactive lectures and group-based activities. It is interesting to note Bartram and Bailey's (2009) findings that students described effective teaching in terms of teaching skills, teacher attributes, staff–student relationships and teacher knowledge, which mirrors the literature on mentorship that identifies the qualities of the mentor and the relationship as the most important factors.

Personal and philosophical beliefs of lecturers

Kane et al. (2002) conducted an extensive review of research studies on the teaching beliefs and practices of university lecturers, concluding that many of these focused on lecturers' reports of their practice, which were not confirmed by direct observation. They advise that it is important to understand the links between beliefs and practice and use the terms 'espoused theories' and 'theories in use', which will be familiar concepts to healthcare professionals. Lindblom-Ylanne et al. (2006) recognise that lecturers' approaches to teaching are influenced by their personal conceptions of teaching. Teacher-centred (content-centred) approaches focus on the transmission of knowledge, whereas student-centred approaches focus on the facilitation of learning, from a constructivist perspective. They report that approaches to teaching are influenced by the lecturers' discipline and also by the context of the teaching. Kember (2009) describes a project to improve the quality of learning and teaching by encouraging lecturers to promote active student engagement with learning. He reports that many lecturers view themselves as experts in their own disciplines and are teacher-centred and content-orientated in their teaching, which is a potential barrier to implementing student-centred approaches to learning.

Theory X and Theory Y

Biggs and Tang (2007) apply the management theory proposed by McGregor (1960) to learning in Higher Education (HE) (see Table 39.1). Theory X operates on low trust and produces low-risk and low-value outcomes, because it reduces the range of learning opportunities (particularly self-directed learning) and it creates anxiety and cynicism in students. Theory Y, on the other hand, encourages students to take responsibility for their learning and promotes active rather than passive learning; it operates on high trust with high-value outcomes.

Theory Y is consistent with recent work by Professor Ronald Barnett, who proposes that students need to be given freedom to develop throughout their education programmes, advising that 'if we want our students to fly, to become themselves, to take off, to take on the world, we have to let them go' (2007: 70). Barnett (2007) proposes that the role of the lecturer in HE is to inspire students and to provide the pedagogical space for them to engage authentically with educational experiences. He argues that this enables students to take responsibility for their thoughts and actions but acknowledges that there are risks associated with this. He recognises that this approach has implications for the role of the lecturer, who has to relinquish control over learning.

Table 39.1 Application of theories X and Y to Higher Education

Theory	Management application	HE application	Learning climate
Theory X	Workers cannot be trusted	Assumes that students do not want to learn and will cheat if given the opportunity Lecturers do not involve students in decisions about their learning	Based on anxiety Lecturer as expert
Theory Y	Workers can be trusted and give better results if given that trust	Didactic approach assumes that students do best when given freedom Student-centred learning with self and peer assessment Humanistic approach	Based on trust Equal relationship between student and lecturer

Source: Adapted from Biggs and Tang, 2007

Tensions in healthcare education

Although Barnett's philosophy of HE is compelling, it is important to consider that the focus of this book is on healthcare education. It is essential, therefore, to ensure that professional requirements are met, to ensure that practitioners are safe and effective at the point of registration. With a shift in the demands of health and social care, educators also need to ensure that professional education develops autonomous practitioners to meet future as well as current demands (Mailloux, 2006). It is evident that professional education occurs in the context of multiple interests, including professional bodies, government, employers, patients and clients. Eraut (2005) contends that this leads to competing agendas for students on professional programmes with inevitable tensions between prescribed content and the aims to develop critical thinking skills, conceptual understanding and to connect theory and practice.

Creativity and humour in teaching

Tauber and Mester (2007) suggest that lecturers can choose their teaching style and should practise a range of skills, in much the same way that actors practise their performances. They stress the value of enthusiasm in promoting learning, arguing that more enthusiastic teachers are perceived to be more effective teachers. They also advise the creative use of verbal and non-verbal techniques, for example animation in voice and body, and humour. Berk (1996) contends that humour is potentially a very powerful strategy within education and he suggests that it should be used as a planned teaching strategy rather than in an 'ad hoc' manner. He reports that the psychological and physiological effects of humour are well documented, but acknowledges that there is a lack of empirical research into humour and education. Struthers (2008) discusses humour in relation to nursing practice, suggesting that it is an abstract concept that is dependent on the personality traits and cognitive schema of the individual. He cautions that, although it is possible to identify the key ingredients of humour, it is difficult to capture its essence or to teach others to use it effectively. Struthers (2008: 302) offers useful guidelines for the use of humour in nursing practice. These are adapted below to provide guidance for lecturers in healthcare:

- Consider the ethical implications.
- Do not risk offending students – for example regarding ethnicity, religion, sexuality.
- Be cautious about jokes relating to health and safety.
- Using humour in healthcare education is not about being a comedian.
- Laugh with students not at them.
- Be prepared to apologise if you use humour inappropriately.
- Be sensitive to your students' sense of humour.
- Be open to humour directed at you.
- Do not overuse humour – spontaneity and timing are part of its magic.

CASE STUDY

I started the MEd course at the same time as moving from a clinical to an educational role, designing and facilitating simulation and clinical skills sessions for a range of hospital staff (from unqualified to postgraduate medical). I had previous experience of teaching but I had never undergone any formal training. Reflecting upon my teaching style upon starting my course, I am aware that my sessions were very much focused on teaching procedures, that is, management of acutely ill patients. Although the sessions were hands-on for the learners, I assumed the role of 'expert' – 'the font of knowledge'. Participants thought that the simulation was theirs to control but I knew that, by manipulating the manikin and questioning, I could direct the session. This was a comfortable position for me; the scenario would accomplish my outcomes, never straying from my well-walked path.

How has this changed during the course? With increased awareness of my own actions, I now give participants more freedom – allowing them to learn by their own actions (or lack of). I am also more aware of the non-technical side of responses, for example, looking away from the actual procedure, and focusing on their feelings, actions and thinking. Reflection was always important, but this is now continuously encouraged to develop critical thinking and judgement skills. I now also use questioning more appropriately, to explore participants' views rather than to reinforce my own position. This necessitates stepping back from the 'I'm right, you're wrong' position. Having more flexibility in the scenarios may mean that all my outcomes are not reached, but with less technically focused simulation this is not a major issue, because reflection can focus on points to be learned regardless of their source.

Finally, how do I see my teaching styles developing? I hope they will continue to be increasingly student-focused and I am currently exploring virtual simulation and online gaming and platforms for educational use.

CONCLUSION

It is evident that student-centred, facilitative teaching styles are more effective than teacher-centred, didactic teaching styles to promote deep learning for students. However, lecturers and practice educators need to use a range of teaching styles to facilitate the complexities of learning within professional education programmes. They need to be aware of their own personal and philosophical stance in relation to approaches to teaching and to develop a range of teaching styles appropriate to the context of healthcare education.

See also: academic staff development; diversity and equality; humanist learning theories; learning styles; practice teaching; teaching strategies

FURTHER READING

Barnett, R. (2007) *A Will to Learn: Being a Student in an Age of Uncertainty*. Berkshire: Open University Press.
Biggs, J. and Tang, C. (2007) *Teaching for Quality Learning at University*, 3rd edn. Buckingham: Society for Research in Higher Education and Open University Press.

REFERENCES

Barnett, R. (2007) *A Will to Learn: Being a Student in an Age of Uncertainty*. Berkshire: Open University Press.
Bartram, B. and Bailey, C. (2009) 'Different students, same difference? A comparison of UK and international students' understandings of "effective teaching"', *Active Learning in Higher Education*, 10 (2): 172–84. doi: 10.1177/1469787409104903.
Berk, R.A. (1996) 'Student ratings of 10 strategies for using humor in college teaching', *Journal on Excellence in College Teaching*, 7 (3): 71–92.
Biggs, J. and Tang, C. (2007) *Teaching for Quality Learning at University*, 3rd edn. Buckingham: Society for Research in Higher Education and Open University Press.
Eraut, M.([1974]2005) 'Continuity of learning', *Learning in Health and Social Care*, 4 (1): 1–6.
Freire, P. ([1974]2005) *Education for Critical Consciousness*. New York: Continuum.
Jarvis, P. (2006) *The Theory and Practice of Teaching*, 2nd edn. London: Routledge.
Kane, R., Sandretto, S. and Heath, C. (2002) 'Telling half the story: a critical review of research on the teaching beliefs and practices of university academics', *Review of Educational Research*, 72(2): 177–228.
Kember, D. (2009) 'Promoting student-centred forms of learning across an entire university', *Higher Education*, 58: 1–13. doi:10.1007/s10734-008-9177-6.
Lindblom-Ylanne, S., Trigwell, K., Nevgi, A. and Ashwin, P. (2006) 'How approaches to teaching are affected by discipline and teaching context', *Studies in Higher Education*, 31 (3): 285–98. doi: 10.1080/03075070600680539.

Mailloux, C.G. (2006) 'The extent to which students' perceptions of faculties' teaching strategies, students' context and perceptions of learner empowerment predict perceptions of autonomy in BSN students', *Nurse Education Today*, 26: 578–85.

McGregor, D.(1960) *The Human Side of Enterprise*. New York: McGraw–Hill.

Sander, P., Stevenson, K., King, M. and Coates, D. (2000) 'University students' expectation of teaching', *Studies in Higher Education*, 25 (3): 309–23.

Struthers, J. (2008) 'Sense of humour', in E. Mason-Whitehead, A. McIntosh, A. Bryan and T. Mason (eds), *Key Concepts in Nursing*. London: Sage. pp. 298–303.

Tauber, R.T. and Mester, T.S. (2007) *Acting Lessons for Teachers: Using Performance Skills in the Classroom*, 2nd edn. Westport, CT: Praeger.

40 transformative learning

Julie Bailey-McHale

DEFINITION

Transformative learning reflects a view of learning that regards the learner holistically and emphasises the continued critical review of one's taken-for-granted assumptions about the world. Mezirow, one of the key writers associated with this concept, describes this as 'transformations in habits of mind' (Mezirow, 2000:17). The means through which this transformation happens is via critical reflection either by the individual or facilitated by another. This type of learning needs to take place within an atmosphere characterised by mutual respect and trust.

KEY POINTS

- Transformative learning is embedded in critical reflection.
- Learning that transforms requires careful selection of specific teaching strategies and an atmosphere of mutual respect.
- By its very nature transformative learning is political.

DISCUSSION

The nature of transformative learning is explored here, particularly in relation to critical reflection. The characteristics associated with the process of this type of learning will be highlighted along with the implications for teaching methods. The political nature of transformative learning will also be identified and discussed.

There is a close relationship between transformative learning and critical reflection. A key feature of this relationship is the importance of understanding the self in relation to multi-contextual situations. Heron (1992) provides a useful framework in which reflection and extended ways of knowing are described and argues that an individual displays four modes of functioning. These are described as: the affective mode, which involves feelings and emotions; the imaginal mode, involving intuition and memory; the conceptual mode, which incorporates reflection and discrimination; and finally the practical mode, which involves intention and action. Heron (1992) goes on to argue that these four modes are then translated into fours ways of knowing. These are:

- experiential: this is evident when engaging with a person, a plan or process.
- presentational: this is evident when an individual understands and appreciates various art forms.
- propositional: this is evident in intellectual activity based on logic and evidence.
- practical: this is evident in the exercising of a skill.

The work of both Heron (1992) and Mezirow (1991, 2000) posits the importance of situated learning, suggesting the imperative of the creation of meaning within a situation. For those involved in self reflection, or facilitating critical reflection in others, attending to meaning or thoughts becomes essential. Mezirow's (2000) assertion that transformative learning is produced through changes in habits of mind is reflected in this. Transformative learning through critical reflection allows the individual to challenge concepts of reality by emphasising that reality is constructed through the interpretation of a situation. And so reality can be changed. This is a crucial aspect of cognitive behavioural therapy (CBT) and the similarity of the work of Mezirow (2000) and Aaron Beck (Beck et al.,1979), the founding father of modern CBT, is evident. Beck et al. (1979) suggested that thoughts are not reality, but that they merely create reality and change occurs when an individual is able to critically analyse alternative explanations and create a new reality. The concept of praxis becomes important in relation to this as the process of action and reflection both promotes understanding and facilitates change. Freire proclaims 'to speak a true word is to transform the world' (1996: 68).

A criticism of Mezirow's work is the emphasis on the self and the assumption of rationality. Scott (2003) highlights the social nature of transformative learning and suggests an individual goes through five stages in the process of transformative learning. These stages are: disequilibrium; internalisation; relationships; imagination; and consciousness. Mezirow (2000) argues that transformative learning can occur gradually over a longer period of time, producing revisions to one's way of understanding phenomena, or that it can also happen in a dramatic manner, producing a significant shift in an individual's view of the world. Both writers, however, suggest that transformative learning is initiated by a dilemma that creates a state of disequilibrium, potentially producing a transformation within the individual and potentially affecting their social world.

Fostering transformative learning is a challenge to the healthcare educator. Key writers agree that the relationship between the learner and the educator is important, particularly the negotiation of power relationships (Freire, 1996; Mezirow, 2000). The need for mutual respect and the nurturing of an atmosphere of trust is essential. The political nature of transformative learning can be seen in the assertion that a neutral education process does not exist (Freire, 1996). The work of Freire describes how education either produces conformity or it challenges the status quo. The philosophical stance of the educator is seen as essential particularly in fostering the mutuality of the learning situation and the need to strive for democratic relationships within the educational setting (Freire, 1996). Yorks and Sharoff (2001) suggest there has been a shift in professional education curricula, particularly in nursing. They argue that nursing has moved away from a reliance on the transfer of knowledge to a recognition of the nurse as a whole person and, importantly, an active agent in his or her own learning. Arguably, this philosophical stance has more potential to create transformative learning situations rather than a reliance on accumulation of knowledge, which Freire (1973, 1996) describes as banking education.

A number of teaching methods are appropriate when considering facilitating critical reflection and transformative learning. Certainly the use of journals can be helpful as can the writing of reflections on critical incidents. A further method, and one generally under-utilised, is the use of drawings or poetry to express emotions or thoughts that may otherwise be difficult to articulate. The process through which learning takes place is also essential; the *way* something is learnt is just as important as *what* is learnt. The emphasis upon the nature of the relationship becomes an important aspect of teaching and learning.

CASE STUDY

Frank is a staff nurse on a surgical ward. He has been qualified for two years and describes himself as a competent and confident nurse. During a night shift Frank was caring for a patient with a number of complex problems. On completion of the Early Warning Score (EWS) documentation, Frank realised the patient was starting to deteriorate and so needed to be reviewed by the doctor on call. Frank bleeped the doctor on call and discussed the details of the patient with him. The doctor was reluctant to come and see the patient, despite Frank referring to the hospital policy regarding such situations. Ultimately the doctor refused to come and review the patient, and suggested that Frank continued to monitor the situation closely. The patient's condition continued to deteriorate and the doctor was bleeped again and requested to attend the ward. On this occasion the doctor came to the ward and examined the patient, was not concerned about the patient's condition and left, with no treatment or interventions prescribed. Monitoring of the patient showed further deterioration and Frank eventually decided to contact the consultant on call and described the situation to her. The consultant agreed to contact the on-call doctor and discuss the case. After a short period of time the on-call doctor returned to the ward and the patient was eventually transferred to the intensive care unit. Frank was extremely upset about the incident and wondered why he had not been more assertive with the on-call doctor.

This led him to reflect upon his own assumptions about the professional roles of the nurse and doctor. He realised, after discussion in his supervision session, that he felt the doctor had superior knowledge to his own and so should not be challenged. On further examination of the situation it was revealed that the doctor was very new to surgery; in fact, he had been in post for only two weeks. It was possible, however, that he had negated the advice of Frank due to his own assumptions about nurses. Frank began to recognise, on a day-to-day basis, further examples of the inappropriate use of power amongst healthcare professionals within the surgical directorate and began to challenge these taken-for-granted assumptions about professional relationships. He began to see his own role as one of advocating for the potentially vulnerable patient and he acknowledged his responsibility for continually developing his skills and knowledge to ensure he could do this effectively. As a result of his reflections, and the change in his beliefs about professional roles, Frank volunteered to teach the new doctors and felt much more confident about his position within the team.

CONCLUSION

The concept of transformative learning is an essential aspect of critical reflection. The central premise of exploring taken-for-granted assumptions and from this exploration creating new ways of understanding the world is a key element of transformative learning. This learning will potentially challenge the status quo in any given situation and give the opportunity to create new meaning. The role of the educator is to create the situations in which this type of learning can be facilitated; this will occur as a result of careful selection of specific teaching and facilitation strategies and also from the ways in which the relationship between the learner and educator is constructed.

See also: humanist learning theories; reflection; teaching strategies

FURTHER READING

Mezirow, J. (2000). 'Learning to think like an adult', in J. Mezirow (ed.), *Learning as Transformation: Critical Perspectives on a Theory in Progress*. San Francisco, CA: Jossey–Bass. pp. 3–33.

REFERENCES

Beck, A., Rush, J., Shaw, B. and Emery, G. (1979) *Cognitive Therapy of Depression*. New York: Guildford Press.

Freire, P. (1973) *Education for Critical Consciousness*. New York: Seabury.

Freire, P. (1996) *Pedagogy of the Oppressed*. Harmondsworth: Penguin.

Heron, J. (1992) *Feeling and Personhood: Psychology in Another Key*. Beverly Hills, CA: Sage.

Mezirow, J. (1991) *Transformative Dimensions of Adult Learning*. San Francisco, CA: Jossey–Bass.

Mezirow, J. (2000) 'Learning to think like an adult', in J. Mezirow (ed.), *Learning as Transformation: Critical Perspectives on a Theory in Progress*. San Francisco, CA: Jossey–Bass. pp. 3–33.

Scott, S. (2003) 'The social construction of transformation', *Journal of Transformative Education*, 1 (3): 264–84.

Yorks, L. and Sharoff, L. (2001) 'An extended epistemology for fostering transformative learning in holistic nursing education and practice', *Holistic Nursing Practice*, 16 (1): 21–9.

transformative learning